ALL ABOUT
BIRTH
CONTROL

Books by Planned Parenthood Federation of America, Inc.:

The Planned Parenthood Women's Health Encyclopedia

All About Sex: A Family Resource on Sex and Sexuality

ALL ABOUT BIRTH CONTROL

A Personal Guide

by Jon Knowles

and Marcia Ringel

Three Rivers Press
New York

Copyright © 1998 by Planned Parenthood Federation of America, Inc.

All rights reserved. No part of this book may be reproduced or transmitted in any form or by any means, electronic or mechanical, including photocopying, recording, or by any information storage and retrieval system, without permission from the publisher.

Published by Three Rivers Press, a division of Crown Publishers, Inc., 201 East 50th Street, New York, New York 10022. Member of the Crown Publishing Group.

Random House, Inc. New York, Toronto, London, Sydney, Auckland www.randomhouse.com

Three Rivers Press and colophon are trademarks of Crown Publishers, Inc.

Printed in the United States of America

Design by Jerry O'Brien

Library of Congress Cataloging-in-Publication Data is available upon request.

ISBN 0-517-88506-9

10   9   8   7   6   5   4   3   2   1

First Edition

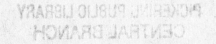

This book is dedicated to the memory and legacy of
Margaret Higgins Sanger, American hero and visionary,
and to all the inspired women and men who have dedicated
themselves to continuing her life's work.

Contents

ACKNOWLEDGMENTS

Authors
Jon Knowles and Marcia Ringel

Planned Parenthood Federation of America Staff
Gloria Feldt, President
Michael S. Burnhill, M.D., D.M.Sc., Vice President for Medical Affairs
Karla Buitrago, editorial Associate/Production Coordinator
Dara Klassel, Director of Legal Affairs
Wendy Lund, Vice President for Marketing
Jon Knowles, Director of Sexual Health Information
Cathy Motamed, Marketing Assistant
Eve Paul, Esq., General Counsel
Barbara Snow, Vice President for Executive Affairs
Kate Thomsen, Director of Medical Affairs

Illustrations: Jim Silks
Condom use illustration: Jon Knowles
Charts: Curtis Tow

Special Thanks
To the National Medical Committee of Planned Parenthood
Federation of America and the nationwide family of Planned
Parenthood medical professionals whose continuing contributions to
the review of our materials and the understanding of contraception
and family planning have made this book possible.

Editorial Coordination and Production
by the People's Medical Society
Charles B. Inlander, President
Karla Morales, Vice President of Editorial Services

Bill Betts, copy editor
Jerry O'Brien, book design
Nancy Rutman, proofer
Sally Lutz, indexer

Preface

There was a time, not too long ago, when Planned Parenthood was the only friend a woman had for information about birth control. Since 1916, Planned Parenthood has served millions of women and men who want to be able to decide when and whether to have a child—women and men who believe that every child should be wanted and loved. Dedicating itself to the health and well-being of women and their families, Planned Parenthood set the standard for women's health care in America and led the movement to ensure reproductive rights and access to reproductive health care. This book is the culmination of that experience.

This book will provide you with current and comprehensive information about all your contraceptive options—including emergency contraception, one of the best-kept secrets in America. It will provide you with information about how each method works, its advantages and disadvantages, side effects, risks, safety, effectiveness, cost, and noncontraceptive health benefits.

The following chapters describe reversible, permanent, and emergency methods of contraception that can help you plan your family and your life. We've included a short chapter on pregnancy options. It may be useful for women who are faced with unintended pregnancy.

Planned Parenthood offers you this book to guide you in your most private choices and to provide you with information about the public and political conflicts that challenge your right to privacy and your right to choose.

We hope this book will help guide you to the family planning choices that suit you best and that sustain your health and well-being.

How Birth Control Changed the Lives of Women and Their Families

In 1965, the U.S. Supreme Court declared in *Griswold v. Connecticut* that married couples had a constitutional right to use contraception in order to plan their families. *Griswold* laid the groundwork for a chain of historic rulings on reproductive freedom—including the 1973 U.S. Supreme Court decision in *Roe v. Wade* that made abortion safe and legal.

Since *Griswold* and its legal offspring, American women and their families have benefited profoundly from the use of family planning. According to the National Center for Health Statistics, the health benefits of *Griswold* were dramatic and immediate. Between 1965 and 1992, the maternal death rate declined more than 75 percent—from 31.6 to 7.8 for every 100,000 live births. During the same period, the deaths of infants under one year of age dropped 60 percent, from 24.7 to 8.5 for every 100,000 live births, and the number of unwanted pregnancies decreased by nearly one-half—from 21 percent of all births to 12 percent.

Access to birth control did much more than save lives during childbirth and infancy. Not only did maternal and infant death rates plummet, but the ability of women to control their fertility also vastly improved their emotional health and that of their families. With the fundamental changes that birth control brought, all families became better equipped to plan for their futures. The gap between the number of children desired and the number born narrowed for couples in every income bracket.

Contraception, once obtainable only on the black market, is now affordable and accessible to nearly all Americans. According to researchers at The Alan Guttmacher Institute, more than 90 percent of couples in the United States have practiced birth control—at least some of the time. The impact worldwide has also been dramatic. In 1950, only one of every eight couples in the world used birth control. Today half of all the couples in the world use some method of contraception.

Contraception Increases Opportunities for All Women

Contraception has lifted women from poverty and helped them manage their lives and plan their futures. By enabling women to make choices about their fertility, access to contraception broadens women's ability to make choices about other aspects of their lives, increasing their capacity to pursue opportunities in education and employment. Since 1965, the number of women in the American labor force has more than doubled, and their income constitutes a growing proportion of family income. The U.S. Bureau of Labor Statistics reports that, in 1965, 25.1 million women were employed outside the home. By 1995, that number had risen to 57.5 million. In a 1994 Harris Poll, more than half of all employed women said they provided at least half of their household income. Access to contraception also allows unmarried women to maintain their independence and pursue their dreams and goals.

Just as birth control has economic benefits for individual women and their families, it also provides economic savings for the health care system. One study in the 1995 *American Journal of Public Health* demonstrated that birth control saves the health care system $9,000 to $14,000 per woman for every five years of use. The cost of regular contraception, including the most expensive methods, is much less than the public and private costs of unintended pregnancies that end in childbirth or abortion.

Birth Control Provides Noncontraceptive Health Benefits

Birth control saves the lives of women and their children. Some forms of contraception also help prevent endometriosis, pelvic inflammatory disease, ectopic pregnancy, and at least two kinds of cancer. Some methods offer protection against sexually transmitted infections and infertility; others reduce the chances of a variety of discomforts, from menstrual irregularity to acne.

For example, the average woman who has ever used the Pill is less likely to die as a result of cancer than a woman who has never used the Pill. In fact, women in their late 40s and 50s who have been long-term users have fewer breast cancers than those who have never used the Pill.

Contraception decreases the number of unwanted births. While many unintended pregnancies lead to wanted births, many do not. According to studies in Europe and in the United States, unwanted childbearing has a negative impact on mothers, couples, families—and most of all, on unwanted children themselves. These studies show that unwanted children suffer emotional, educational, and functional disorders that worsen as they reach adulthood, even if they are born to healthy, adult women who have stable marriages and adequate financial resources.

Wanted children are happier and more successful in life than unwanted children. Children who are born wanted are less likely to be emotionally disabled throughout their lives. Although they are no more intelligent than unwanted children, they are far more able to live up to their intellectual capabilities. They are more likely to enjoy school, get higher grades, and appear intelligent to their parents, teachers, and classmates, and they are more than twice as likely as unwanted children to pursue higher education.

These studies also show that wanted children seem to suffer less physical abuse, parental neglect, malnourishment, and abandonment. They are half as likely as unwanted children to have a record of juvenile delinquency. They are up to four times less likely to have a record of criminal activity and are less likely to abuse alcohol and drugs in youth and early childhood. They are also more likely to postpone sexual activity and have better relationships at school, at work, and with friends, and they tend to have happier marriages.

Unintended Pregnancy Is Still a Problem in the United States

Although access to birth control has reduced the number of unplanned pregnancies in the last 40 years, the National Academy of Sciences reports that the numbers of unintended pregnancies are rising. Currently, more than half of all pregnancies in America continue to be unplanned—American women still experience more than 3 million unintended pregnancies each year. Births from unintended pregnancies had decreased during the 1970s to 37 percent of all births in 1982, according to The Alan Guttmacher Institute. But that trend was reversed during the last 15 years. Currently, 56 percent of all births are from unintended pregnancies, and 44 percent of those are terminated by induced abortion.

The Alan Guttmacher Institute reports that more than half of all unintended pregnancies occur among the 10 percent of reproductive age women who use no contraception. On the other hand, less than half of unintended pregnancies occur among the nearly 90 percent of reproductive age women who *use* contraception.

Unintended pregnancy can be very disturbing for women who experience it. It also has serious public health consequences. According to the National Institutes of Health, women with unintended pregnancies are less likely to seek early prenatal care and are more likely to use harmful substances such as alcohol and tobacco. They are more likely to have immature or premature, low-birth–weight babies.

The National Institutes of Health also reports that American women have more unintended pregnancies than women in other Western democracies, and they have one abortion for every two births. The Alan Guttmacher Institute reports that the rate of abortion in the United States is two to four times higher than that in other Western democracies—even though women in those other nations have easier access to abortion than American women do.

Sterilization, which is intended to be permanent and requires surgery, is the contraceptive choice of more than one-third of all couples. In an era when divorce and remarriage are commonplace, however, sterilization may not be the ideal method of contraception, especially for younger couples. According to the National Institutes of Health, 30 percent of the low-income women who intended to be sterilized did not understand that the procedure would make it nearly impossible for them to have more children. The Alan Guttmacher Institute reports that women 30 to 34 use sterilization, despite its permanence, more than any other method of contraception. It is also used by more than 20 percent of women 25 to 29 years of age.

Clearly, not all American women have found a method of contraception that suits them. The development of more options for reversible contraception may offer women and men more desirable alternatives to permanent surgical methods. Despite the current limitations of contraceptive technology, however, access to existing methods of safe and effective birth control has greatly enhanced American life:

- Women live longer and healthier lives.
- Women can control their lives, their bodies, and their futures.
- More babies are born healthy, cared-for, and loved.
- Families can be relieved of the financial and emotional challenges of supporting more children than they can afford.

The bottom line is that women and their families benefit enormously from family planning through contraception.

Chapter

1

◆

What Is Planned Parenthood?

Planned Parenthood® Federation of America, Inc., is the world's oldest and largest voluntary reproductive health care organization. We believe that everyone has the right to choose when or whether to have a child and that every child should be wanted and loved.

Planned Parenthood affiliates operate more than 900 health centers nationwide. Its 20,000 volunteers and staff members provide medical, educational, and counseling services for millions of people each year.

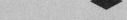

The Planned Parenthood Mission

Planned Parenthood believes in the fundamental right of each individual, throughout the world, to manage his or her fertility—regardless of the individual's income, marital status, race, ethnicity, sexual orientation, age, national origin, or residence. We believe that respect and value for diversity in all aspects of our organization are essential to our well-being. We believe that reproductive self-determination must be voluntary and must preserve an individual's right to privacy. We further believe that such self-determination will contribute to a better quality of life, strong family relationships, and a stable population.

Based on these beliefs, and reflecting the diverse communities in which we operate, the mission of Planned Parenthood is:

- to provide comprehensive reproductive and complementary health care services in settings that preserve and protect the essential privacy and rights of each individual
- to advocate public policies that guarantee these rights and ensure access to such services
- to provide educational programs that enhance understanding of individual and societal implications of human sexuality
- to promote the advancement of technology in reproductive health care and encourage understanding of its inherent ethical, behavioral, and social implications

Margaret Sanger

Planned Parenthood traces its origins to the first birth control clinic in America, founded in 1916 by Margaret Sanger, the American hero who transformed the lives of women around the world by establishing the reproductive rights movement.

Sanger was born in 1879 and grew up in an Irish immigrant family of 11 children in Corning, New York. Working as a nurse on the Lower East Side of New York City, Sanger was deeply moved by the suffering of poor women with large families who were unable to prevent yet another unwanted pregnancy. It was a time when women were expected to bear as many children as possible—even if it made them sick and old before their time and even if it killed them. She decided to do something about it.

On October 16, 1916, in the Brownsville community of Brooklyn, Sanger, with her sister Ethel Byrne and an associate, Fania Mindell, opened the first birth control clinic in America, providing contraceptive advice to desperately poor immigrant women. Less than a month after the clinic opened, all three were arrested for violating federal and local laws that defined contraceptives as "obscene." Sanger refused to pay the fine for her role in the clinic, choosing to spend 30 days in prison. There, she taught birth control to other inmates.

The arrests, and Sanger's stand, galvanized public anger and called attention to the absurdity of the "Comstock laws" that prohibited the distribution of information about sex, sexuality, contraception, and human reproduction. With Sanger's leadership, the birth control movement grew rapidly in size and impact in the next two decades. Sanger gained worldwide renown, respect, and admiration for founding the American birth control movement and, later, the Planned Parenthood Federation of America, as well as for developing and encouraging family planning efforts throughout the world. Sanger's visionary accomplishments as a social reformer have been matched by very few. She convinced the world to embrace principles that were once abhorrent and are now taken for granted. Sanger convinced us that:

- A woman's right to control her body is the foundation of her human rights.
- Every person should be able to decide when or whether to have a child.
- Every child should be wanted and loved.
- Women are as entitled as men to sexual pleasure and fulfillment.

Sanger accomplished her life's mission by bringing about the reversal of federal and state Comstock laws. She helped establish the contemporary American model for the protection of civil rights through nonviolent civil disobedience—a model that later propelled the civil rights, antiwar, women's rights, and AIDS-action movements. When the Rev. Dr. Martin Luther King Jr. was awarded the first Planned Parenthood Federation of America Margaret Sanger Award, he wrote, "Our sure beginning in the struggle for equality by nonviolent direct action may not have been so resolute without the tradition established by Margaret Sanger and people like her."

Sanger created access to birth control for poor, minority, and immigrant women and expanded the American concept of voluntarism and grassroots organizing by setting up a network of volunteer-driven family planning centers across the United States.

In her lifetime, Sanger won the respect of international figures of all races and ethnicities, including the Dr. King, Mahatma Gandhi, Shidzue Kato—the foremost family planning advocate in Japan—and Lady Dhanvanthi Rama Rau of India.

Sanger's accomplishments will never die. Her ideas are here to stay. Women in America must always cherish their right to decide when and whether to have a child, the principle that every child deserves to be wanted and loved, and their equal right to sexual pleasure. Millions of women worldwide agree. Each day of their lives, they live the legacy of Margaret Sanger. She would be very proud.

Until the time of her death in 1966, Sanger continued to exert her influence on the family planning movement and to lend her support to the projects she considered most urgent.

Advances in Reproductive Health in the 1960s

Margaret Sanger was also the driving force behind the development of the Pill—a major step in the development of safe and effective birth control. She avidly supported the development of a "magic pellet"— an inexpensive, medically safe, completely reliable contraceptive that could be taken orally or by injection. Sanger's years of scientific and advocacy efforts, financially supported by her friend Katharine Dexter McCormick, were rewarded in the early 1950s, when Gregory Pincus, M.D., demonstrated that injections of the steroid progesterone could stop ovulation in laboratory animals. In 1960, the U.S. Food and Drug Administration (FDA) approved the sale of oral steroids—the Pill. Shortly thereafter, the first intrauterine devices (IUDs) also became available. The Pill and the IUD heralded major advances both in science and in attitudes about reproductive freedom.

Perhaps the single most important advance in reproductive health in the 1960s, however, was the U.S. Supreme Court decision in *Griswold v. Connecticut*. The decision bears the name of Estelle

Griswold, then the executive director of Planned Parenthood of Connecticut, who was sued by the state for dispensing contraceptives and contraceptive information. The court ruled that laws prohibiting the use of birth control by married couples violated the right of marital privacy.

Advances in Reproductive Health in the 1970s

The most dramatic advance in reproductive rights during the 1970s took place in the midst of a reawakened civil rights movement, the winding down of the war in Vietnam, and the drive for the Equal Rights Amendment. On January 22, 1973, the U.S. Supreme Court handed down its decision in *Roe v. Wade,* striking down restrictive abortion laws throughout the nation and declaring that the U.S. Constitution protects a woman's right, in consultation with her physician, to choose an abortion.

Not surprisingly, the more the family planning movement was absorbed into the mainstream, the more vigorously religious political extremists marshaled their forces. The first anti–choice organizations were launched in several U.S. communities in the 1960s. These local "Right-to-Life" Leagues had the strong support of the Catholic church. In 1973, the *National* Right to Life Committee was organized. Its express purpose was to overturn *Roe v. Wade* and the new state statutes that had made abortion safe and legal.

Challenges to Reproductive Health in the 1980s and 1990s

The opposition to abortion rights disguises a continuing attack on the right to family planning. Many adherents of these anti-choice organizations oppose contraception as well as abortion. They have proposed statutes and constitutional amendments that would outlaw the IUD and some forms of the Pill and severely restrict access to federally funded family planning services. Opposition to contraception within the anti-abortion movement continues to this day.

The well-funded anti-choice minority has become a strong political influence in U.S. politics. Extremist anti-choice factions have turned to terrorism, and efforts to barricade clinics and harass patients and reproductive health care workers have become commonplace. Future historians who look back on the 1980s and 1990s may well regard it as a new era of Comstockery, for not since Margaret Sanger opened the Brownsville clinic have family planning activists had to fight such opposition.

However, the overwhelming majority of Americans continue to believe that individuals should be able to make their own reproductive decisions without government interference. In its 1996 national survey, Planned Parenthood found that 90 percent of Americans agree that it is important to have family planning services, and that 67 percent think it is important to have international family planning services. In a more recent 1997 survey, Planned Parenthood found that 76 percent of Americans favor increasing access to family planning services; 75 percent agree that the number of abortions in the United States would be lower if more people had access to birth control; 76 percent favor increased public funding for family planning services and counseling to reduce the number of unintended pregnancies; 85 percent think it is important for teens to have access to family planning services; 77 percent favor requiring schools to provide sex education, and 63 percent favor requiring insurance companies to cover birth control.

Since Margaret Sanger established her first clinic in Brownsville, the range of services and the number of people served by Planned Parenthood have grown by leaps and bounds. Today, Planned Parenthood serves nearly 5 million women and men in the United States and the developing world. At the close of the century, family planning organizations and the millions of Americans who support reproductive rights are firmly committed to ensuring that the new century will reflect as much progress as the last. Margaret Sanger would be very proud of what her movement has accomplished.

A Continuing Commitment to Family Planning

For 80 years, Planned Parenthood has been in the forefront of the battle for reproductive rights, and the vast majority of Americans continue to uphold its principles. Financial support for Planned Parenthood's national activities and service comes from private sector contributors, including corporations, foundations, affiliates, and 700,000 individual donors. Affiliate activities are funded through private contributions, client fees, corporate and government grants, and third-party reimbursement for services.

The work of Planned Parenthood is guided by national and local volunteer boards of directors and is supported in the implementation of national and international educational, medical, communications, fund-raising, legal, and public affairs programs by staffs headquartered in New York City; Washington, D.C.; San Francisco; and Chicago.

The work of Planned Parenthood is enhanced by its special independent affiliate, The Alan Guttmacher Institute. The institute provides domestic and international research, policy analysis, and public education to help women and men make informed decisions about their reproductive lives.

Planned Parenthood is a leader in the international family planning movement. Through Family Planning International Assistance®, its international division, Planned Parenthood supports nongovernment and government agencies to promote, initiate, maintain, and expand family planning services in Asia and the Pacific, Africa, Latin America, and the Caribbean. Planned Parenthood is also a founding member of the International Planned Parenthood Federation.

A Commitment to Health Care Services

With medical standards, training, and technical assistance provided by the national office, Planned Parenthood affiliates offer a wide range of medical services, counseling, and/or referrals for:

- family planning counseling and birth control
- pregnancy testing and counseling
- gynecological care, Pap tests, and breast exams
- emergency contraception
- HIV testing and counseling
- comprehensive, age-appropriate sexuality education
- screening and treatment for sexually transmitted infections
- infertility screening and counseling
- voluntary sterilization for women and men
- reproductive medical exams for men
- safer-sex counseling
- midlife services
- abortion
- prenatal care
- adoption
- primary health care

You can reach the Planned Parenthood health center nearest you by calling 800-230-PLAN.

Planned Parenthood cooperates with other community and national groups to ensure greater access to family planning and health services and to promote the sexual and reproductive health and well-being of the individual, the family, and the community.

Decades after encouraging development of the Pill, Planned Parenthood continues its tradition of research and development by participating in trials for the medical abortion drugs, methotrexate and mifepristone—the latter known in Europe as RU-486. It is hoped that the use of these medications for safe and legal abortion will soon be approved by the FDA.

A Commitment to Sexuality Education

Planned Parenthood educators form the largest network of professional sexuality educators in the United States. They offer a broad range of educational and training interventions to address the needs of their communities. Affiliate programs to increase sexual literacy and encourage comprehensive and responsible sexuality education are aided by national leadership and support, and include the following:

- programs designed for parents, adolescents, and younger children, enabling them to enhance sexuality learning within the family
- workshops and seminars for human-service providers, including teachers, physicians, nurses, social workers, and clergy
- presentations to civic and business groups and other community organizations on sexual and reproductive issues
- classes for students in grades K–12 to impart information about healthy sexual development and to build decision-making and communication skills

Planned Parenthood health centers offer a wide range of information resources, including pamphlets, books, newsletters, and videotapes on a variety of sexual health topics. In addition, many Planned Parenthood affiliates provide valuable information on the World Wide Web. They can all be reached at http://www.plannedparenthood.org

A Commitment to Advocacy

To ensure universal access to comprehensive family planning information and services, Planned Parenthood engages in national, state, and local programs to:

- alert the public to the threats to civil liberties posed by those who oppose the right of an individual to decide when or whether to have a child
- mobilize the vast majority of Americans who already support the right of individual choice in family planning

With well-coordinated public affairs, legal, communications, and fund-raising efforts, Planned Parenthood demonstrates to key decision-makers that the American public opposes restrictions on the fundamental right to reproductive choice. These activities include the following:

- building networks with other community and national groups
- mobilizing letter-writing drives
- developing advertising and other media campaigns
- engaging in litigation to protect individuals from restrictive legislation
- providing information to the media, religious leaders, other community health and civil rights groups, and concerned individuals
- providing educational information to the public and elected officials
- working to bring new methods of contraception to the United States

Further strengthening our commitment to advocacy, the Planned Parenthood Action Fund:
- encourages and protects informed individual choice regarding reproductive health care
- advocates public policies that guarantee the right to choice and full and nondiscriminatory access to reproductive health care
- fosters and preserves a social and political climate favorable to the exercise of reproductive choice

The Planned Parenthood Action Fund also provides financial and technical assistance to more than 40 local and state Planned Parenthood groups nationwide to enhance their own grassroots lobbying, electoral activity, and public policy work.

All these activities are designed to increase government and private-sector commitment to and understanding of the need for comprehensive family planning services for all who want and need them. Support sexual and reproductive health and rights for women and men worldwide: For more information or an appointment with the Planned Parenthood health center nearest you, call 800-230-PLAN (7526). To order Planned Parenthood publications and products, call 800-669-0156. You can also visit us on the World Wide Web at **http://www.plannedparenthood.org** to learn more about our organization and your sexual health.

2

Reproduction and Contraception— How They Work

- *Women's Reproductive Anatomy and How It Works*
- *The Menstrual Cycle*
- *Men's Reproductive Anatomy and How It Works*
- *How Pregnancy Occurs—Fertilization and Implantation*
- *Contraception and How It Works*

Women and men who understand how their reproductive systems work are able to use contraceptives more effectively than other women and men. Here are the basics for understanding human reproduction and contraception.

Women's Reproductive Anatomy and How It Works

The supporting structure of a woman's internal reproductive system is the **pelvic girdle**—a bony and muscular structure shaped like a basin that supports the internal sex and reproductive organs.

11

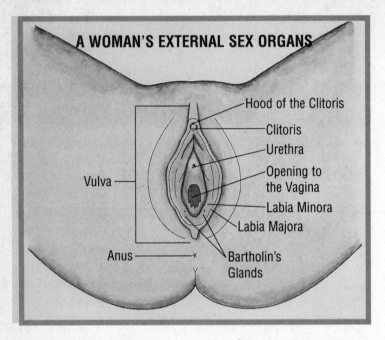

A WOMAN'S EXTERNAL SEX ORGANS

Hood of the Clitoris
Clitoris
Urethra
Opening to the Vagina
Labia Minora
Labia Majora
Vulva
Anus
Bartholin's Glands

A woman's external sex organs are contained in an area called the **vulva.** The external sex organs located in the vulva are the outer lips (labia majora), the inner lips (labia minora), the opening to the vagina, the clitoris, and two Bartholin's glands. Two Skene's glands are located beneath the surface of the vulva on each side of the urethra.

The **clitoris** is an organ that is located in the soft folds of the labia that meet just above the opening of the urethra. The clitoris swells during excitement and is a source of sexual pleasure when stimulated. The clitoris varies in size from woman to woman, but it is often about the size of a pea.

The **Bartholin's** and **Skene's glands** secrete fluids that provide lubrication during sexual excitement. The Bartholin's glands are located on each side of the opening to the vagina. The Skene's glands are located just within the opening to the urethra on each side of the urethra.

The **urethra** is located in the vulva just below the clitoris and above the opening to the vagina. It is not part of the reproductive sys-

A WOMAN'S INTERNAL REPRODUCTIVE ORGANS

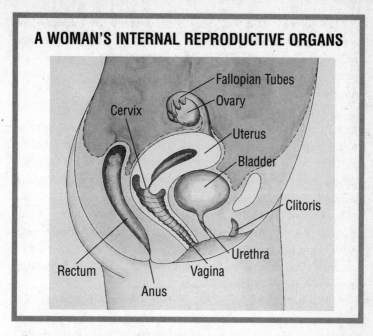

tem. Urine from the bladder passes through the urethra and leaves the body through the opening of the urethra. The **anus** is located behind the vulva. It is the opening from the rectum (lower intestine). Solid waste leaves the body through the anus.

The vulva is connected to a woman's internal reproductive system by the vagina. A woman's internal reproductive organs include two ovaries, two fallopian tubes, the uterus, the cervix, and the vagina. The **vagina** is a stretchable passage between a woman's vulva and her cervix and uterus. It is four to five inches long. The vagina opens onto the vulva and is surrounded by a constrictor muscle. The penis enters the vagina during vaginal intercourse. The vagina is also the birth canal.

The upper end of the vagina contains the **cervix,** the narrow lower portion (or neck) of the uterus. About one-half of the cervix projects into the vagina. The opening of the cervix into the vagina is called the mouth of the cervix. At its narrowest point, the opening of the cervix is about as wide as the lead in a pencil.

The **uterus** is commonly known as the womb. The interior of the uterus is a narrow, triangle-shaped cavity lined by the endometrium and surrounded by thick muscular walls. During pregnancy, the embryo and fetus develop in the uterus. The muscles of the uterus contract during labor to deliver the fetus from the uterus.

The **fallopian tubes** extend from the top of each side of the uterus. Each fallopian tube ends near an ovary. The outer edge of each tube has fine hairlike fringes called cilia that sweep a mature egg from the ovary into the tube. The contractions of the fallopian tube and the movements of the cilia move the egg toward the uterus.

Each **ovary** is attached by ligaments to the side of the uterus and to the walls of the pelvis. The ovaries produce the hormones estrogen and progesterone, as well as a small amount of testosterone. Every ovary has thousands of follicles, tiny sacs that each hold an immature egg. Women are born with 30,000 to 200,000 follicles in each ovary. The follicle grows as an egg matures.

The **egg** (ovum) is the female reproductive cell. Full of nourishment to sustain a growing preembryo in its first few days, the egg is the largest human cell. It is about the size of the dot of a newsprint "i."

The Menstrual Cycle

The menstrual cycle is a pattern of fertility and infertility that usually repeats itself monthly. Menstruation begins at puberty and ends with menopause. The menstrual cycle may last from 21 to 35 days. The length of the cycle is different for each woman and may also change from month to month.

Here are the key terms related to a woman's fertility pattern:

- **Ovulation.** The release of an egg from an ovary.
- **Hormone.** A natural chemical carried in the bloodstream that influences how glands and organs work. The four hormones that regulate the menstrual cycle are progesterone, estrogen, LH (luteinizing hormone), and FSH (follicle-stimulating hormone).

- **Pituitary gland.** A small gland located at the base of the brain that releases hormones that influence how the body and menstrual cycle work.
- **Follicle.** A tiny sac that holds a single egg. Women are born with 30,000 to 200,000 follicles in each ovary. The follicle grows as an egg matures.
- **Menstruation.** The flow of blood, fluid, and uterine lining tissue (endometrium) out of the uterus through the vagina. Menstruation occurs every 21 to 35 days and lasts from three to seven days. After menstruation, a new endometrium grows in the uterus. The lining will break down and flow out of the uterus again in accordance with a woman's cycle unless pregnancy has occurred.

The menstrual cycle can be divided into two parts: before ovulation and after ovulation. During the first half of the menstrual cycle, three major steps occur:

- Menstruation takes place, usually from Day 1 to Day 5.
- An egg matures in the follicle of an ovary. The maturing is caused by the release of FSH from the pituitary gland between Day 5 and Day 7.
- The lining of the uterus begins to thicken. This is caused by the release of estrogen from the follicle between Day 7 and Day 11.

At ovulation, the ripe egg is released from the follicle. Ovulation is triggered by the release of LH from the pituitary gland about 14 days before the start of the next menstrual cycle.

During the second half of the menstrual cycle, three more major steps occur:

- The ripe egg is swept into the fallopian tube and travels toward the uterus.
- After ovulation, the follicle releases progesterone and estrogen, causing further thickening of the lining of the uterus.
- If pregnancy does not take place, the follicle stops producing estrogen and progesterone, which causes the lining to break down and flow out of the uterus.

Men's Reproductive Anatomy and How It Works

The external sex organs of men are the penis and scrotum. The internal reproductive organs include two testes, two seminal vesicles, two Cowper's glands, and the prostate gland. The glands are connected by tubes called the epididymides, vasa deferentia, and urethra.

The **scrotum** is a sac of skin divided into two parts, each of which holds one testis, one epididymis, and a portion of one vas def-

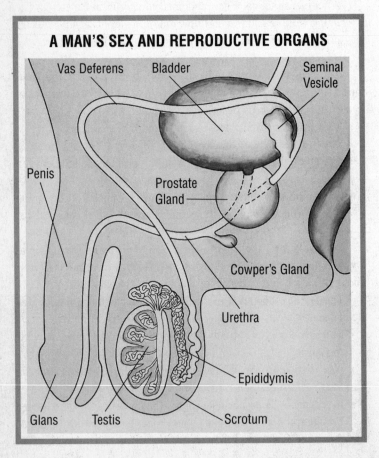

A MAN'S SEX AND REPRODUCTIVE ORGANS

Vas Deferens · Bladder · Seminal Vesicle · Penis · Prostate Gland · Cowper's Gland · Urethra · Epididymis · Glans · Testis · Scrotum

erens. The scrotum keeps the testes up to 5°F cooler than normal body temperature in order to allow for production of sperm. The scrotum also protects the testes from injury.

The **testes,** also called testicles, are two ball-like glands inside the scrotum. Within them, a network of tiny tubes constantly produces sperm. Sperm mature in the **epididymides,** tubes that are tightly coiled over the top and behind each testis. Sperm are carried from each epididymis to the seminal vesicles through a long, narrow tube called the vas deferens. (The plural of vas deferens is vasa deferentia.)

The **seminal vesicles,** located beneath the bladder, produce seminal fluid in which sperm move and are nourished. Seminal fluid combined with secretions from the prostate and Cowper's glands is called semen.

The **prostate gland** is also located beneath the bladder. The prostate gland produces a thin, alkaline fluid that helps sperm move. The fluid also neutralizes the acid in a man's urethra and a woman's vagina.

The **urethra** is a tube that runs from the bladder to the opening in the glans of the penis. The urethra carries urine from the bladder and semen from the vasa deferentia.

The two **Cowper's glands** are attached to the urethra as it descends from the prostate gland. The Cowper's glands secrete the fluid that makes the seminal fluid sticky.

The **penis** is formed of spongy tissue that fills with blood and becomes erect during sexual excitement. A man can ejaculate semen from his penis into a woman's vagina during vaginal intercourse.

The **glans** is the soft tip of the penis. In uncircumcised men, the foreskin covers the glans when the penis is soft. The glans is highly sensitive—equivalent to the clitoris of a woman as a source of sexual pleasure.

The **foreskin** is a retractable tube of skin that covers and protects the glans of the penis. With circumcision the foreskin is removed.

Sperm are the reproductive cells in men. Sperm are produced in the testes and mature in the epididymides. Mature sperm move from the epididymides into the vasa deferentia. During sexual excitement, the vasa deferentia and the other internal reproductive organs tighten and relax in a pulselike rhythm. The contractions push the sperm through the vasa deferentia into the urethra.

In the urethra, fluids from the prostate gland, seminal vesicles, and Cowper's glands mix to form **semen.** The semen is pushed through the urethra by the pulselike contractions of all the internal reproductive organs.

At the peak of sexual excitement, the semen spurts out of the opening of the urethra in the glans of the penis. This is called ejaculation. The liquid that oozes out of the penis during sexual excitement before ejaculation is called pre-ejaculate.

How Pregnancy Occurs: Fertilization and Implantation

Fertilization is the union of egg and sperm. When implantation occurs, pregnancy begins. Knowing how fertilization and implantation happen helps increase understanding of how birth control works.

Here are the key terms related to fertilization and implantation:

- **Vaginal intercourse.** The penis is inserted in the vagina. If ejaculation takes place, semen is deposited at the opening of the cervix.
- **Fertilization.** This occurs when one sperm penetrates an egg.
- **Preembryo.** This is the term used for the ball of cells that develops after fertilization until about five days after implantation, when it becomes an embryo.
- **Implantation.** The preembryo embeds in the lining of the uterus. Pregnancy begins.

The menstrual cycle prepares the body for pregnancy in the following ways:

- Menstruation occurs. The old uterine lining clears away so a new one can grow.
- An egg matures in the follicle. The lining of the uterus thickens and prepares to receive the fertilized egg.

- At ovulation, the mature egg is released and swept into the fallopian tube.

Fertilization usually occurs in the outer one-third of the fallopian tube. Throughout the menstrual cycle, intercourse is most likely to result in fertilization during three consecutive time periods:

- Before ovulation. Sperm can live up to seven days in the fallopian tubes. If the egg is released during that time, fertilization can

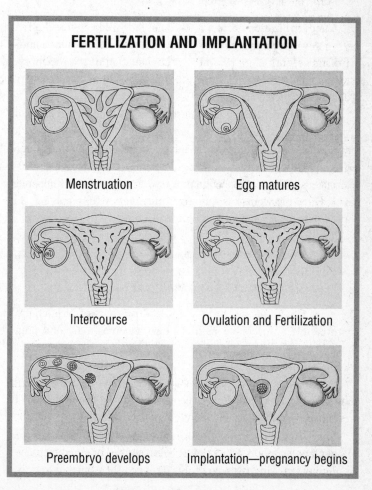

FERTILIZATION AND IMPLANTATION

Menstruation

Egg matures

Intercourse

Ovulation and Fertilization

Preembryo develops

Implantation—pregnancy begins

take place. Fertilization usually occurs during the six days end-
ing in ovulation.

- At ovulation. The egg is ready to be fertilized within two hours
  after it is released from the follicle. If vaginal intercourse occurs
  during this time, fertilization is also likely to result.
- After ovulation. An egg may live a day or so after its release
  from the follicle. If vaginal intercourse occurs within this time,
  fertilization is less likely but may also result.

After fertilization occurs, it takes the fertilized egg three to five
days to move down the fallopian tube. As it travels, it divides a number of times, forming a preembryo. Implantation of the preembryo
usually takes place in the upper portion of the uterine lining and is
probably completed about nine days after fertilization.

When pregnancy begins, menstrual cycles and ovulation stop.
Progesterone and estrogen continue to be produced by the follicle
that released the egg (corpus luteum) in order to maintain the uterine lining while the embryo grows into a fetus. The presence of progesterone also stops the ovulation process for the duration of the pregnancy. Once the woman is no longer pregnant or fully nursing, the
normal pattern of the menstrual cycle resumes.

Contraception and How It Works

There are many kinds of birth control. Most kinds of birth control
are reversible. A reversible method allows a woman to become pregnant when she and her partner stop using it. All reversible methods
are available to teenagers without a parent's permission.

Some kinds of birth control are permanent. Permanent birth
control, or sterilization, is not recommended for young people. It
prevents people from having children afterward.

Some kinds of reversible birth control are available in drugstores
without a prescription. Others must be prescribed or fitted by a doctor or clinician. Most birth control is designed for women to use.

All birth control methods are intended to prevent pregnancy in one or more of the following ways:

- by preventing the sperm from meeting the egg
- by keeping ovaries from releasing eggs
- by preventing fertilized eggs from implanting in the lining of the uterus

Preventing Fertilization

There are many ways to prevent the sperm from meeting the egg. The surest way is not to have vaginal intercourse. Some men and women choose to abstain from all kinds of sex play. This is called abstinence or celibacy. Other women and men abstain from vaginal intercourse but enjoy various other kinds of sex play. This is called outercourse. Many people abstain from sexual intercourse until they are past their teens. Some wait until they are married. Some choose never to have sexual intercourse at all.

Many people use withdrawal as a method of contraception when no other method is available. Withdrawal means that the man must pull his penis out of the vagina before he ejaculates. But it doesn't always prevent pregnancy because men leak a few drops of pre-ejaculate before they ejaculate. Even these few drops can cause pregnancy. Also, many men become so sexually excited that they don't withdraw in time.

Some women and their partners try to predict their fertility patterns. Those that practice periodic abstinence keep very careful records to try to predict when pregnancy might happen and abstain from vaginal intercourse whenever they think there's a chance it could cause pregnancy. Others have intercourse but use other birth control methods during those times.

Male and female condoms and contraceptive foams, creams, jellies, and suppositories are all methods that prevent fertilization by forming barriers to prevent the sperm from entering the fallopian tubes. They can be bought over the counter—that is, without a prescription—because they rarely have side effects when used as directed. Male condoms are worn on the penis. Female condoms, foams, creams, jellies, and suppositories are inserted into the vagina before vaginal intercourse.

Cervical caps and diaphragms also form barriers that prevent the sperm from entering the fallopian tubes and joining with the egg. Cervical caps and diaphragms are worn in the vagina before, during, and after vaginal intercourse. They are available only by prescription. Intrauterine devices (IUDs), also available by prescription, also prevent fertilization. IUDs are inserted into the uterus and work continuously for up to 10 years.

Sterilization is a permanent kind of birth control usually chosen by older people who are very sure they will not want any children in the future. Men and women who choose sterilization have a simple operation to keep eggs and sperm from meeting. In tubal sterilization, the fallopian tubes are blocked to keep sperm from meeting with the egg. In vasectomy, the vasa deferentia are blocked to keep sperm from meeting with the egg.

Preventing Ovulation

The Pill, Depo-Provera®, and Norplant® usually work by preventing ovulation. They can also thicken cervical mucus to prevent fertilization. Birth control pills require a prescription and are taken daily on a monthly schedule. IUDs may also prevent ovulation. Depo-Provera is injected into the arm or buttocks every 12 weeks. Norplant is inserted under the skin of the arm and lasts for five years. Prescription birth control, like many other prescription drugs and devices, may have side effects and health risks for some women.

Women who breast-feed during the day and night for the first six months after giving birth may also prevent ovulation—if they fully breast-feed. This means they must breast-feed every four hours during the day and every six hours during the night and must not supplement breast milk with any other nourishment for their babies. This method of contraception is called the lactational amenorrhea method (LAM).

Preventing Implantation

In the rare circumstance that fertilization occurs during the use of the Pill, Depo-Provera, Norplant, or an IUD, these methods are likely to prevent implantation of the fertilized egg.

Contraceptive Choices in the United States

More than 60 percent of women between ages 15 and 44 use some method of contraception. Nearly 26 percent of them rely on tubal sterilization. More than 10 percent are protected by their partner's vasectomy. The Pill is the most commonly used reversible method of contraception in America—it is used by nearly 25 percent of women who are at risk for unintended pregnancy. The male condom is used by the partners of about 19 percent of women at risk of unintended pregnancy. Nearly 3 percent use injectables. A similar number uses withdrawal. More than 2 percent use periodic abstinence, and nearly 2 percent use the diaphragm. More than 1 percent use implants. Fewer than 1 percent now use the IUD. And fewer than 1 percent use the female condom.

Having vaginal intercourse without birth control, even once, even the first time, can cause pregnancy. Of every 100 sexually active women who don't use birth control in the course of a year, 85 will become pregnant.

Every woman and man must choose the methods that best suit them. The following chapter offers some information about the considerations they may make in order to decide which method to choose.

Choosing a Method of Birth Control

- *How Reversible Will the Method Be?*
- *How Effective Will the Method Be?*
- *How Safe Will the Method Be?*
- *Will the Method Protect Against Sexually Transmitted Infections (STIs)?*
- *How Affordable and Available Will the Method Be?*
- *How Well Will a Contraceptive Method Fit into a Person's Lifestyle?*
- *How Private Does the Method Need to Be?*

People's contraceptive needs change throughout their lives. To decide which method to use, they consider how well each one will work for them.

How Reversible Will the Method Be?

Most younger women and men who choose to use contraception want to be able to have children at some future time in their lives. They want to protect themselves against unintended pregnancy now, but they also want to be able to reverse the contraceptive effects when they decide they want to have a child.

Reversibility, on the other hand, may not be desired by women and men who have completed their families or who know they do not want any children. They may want a permanent method—either tubal sterilization for women or vasectomy for men.

Permanent methods are appropriate for mature women and men who know that:

- They want to enjoy having sex without causing pregnancy.
- They don't want to have a child in the future.
- Their partners agree that their families are complete and no more children are wanted.
- They and their partners have concerns about the side effects of other methods.
- Other methods are unacceptable.
- The woman's health would be threatened by a future pregnancy.
- They don't want to pass on a hereditary illness or disability.
- They are men who choose vasectomy to spare their partners the surgery and expense of tubal sterilization, which is more complicated and costly.

Permanent methods are not appropriate for women or men if:

- They want to have a child in the future.
- They are being pressured to choose permanent methods by their partners, friends, or family.
- They have marriage or sexual problems, *short-term* mental or physical illnesses, financial worries, or are out of work. Permanent methods are not good solutions for *temporary* problems such as these.
- They have not considered possible changes in their lives such as divorce, remarriage, or the death of a child.

Many couples may prefer a method that is quickly and easily reversible. All barrier methods of birth control, behavioral methods of birth control, and the IUD are immediately reversible. Fertility is restored to its previous levels as soon as the contraceptive method is discontinued. Hormonal methods, however, are not reversible right away because it takes time for a hormone to leave the system. Women who are considering a hormonal method and are planning to become pregnant soon must be sure to know how much time is needed to reverse the contraceptive effects of the methods they are considering.

If a woman and a man want to have a child after a period of contraceptive use, it is especially important for them to protect themselves from STIs during the time they are using whatever contraceptive method they have chosen. Many of these infections have no symptoms or do not have symptoms until the latter stages, and with time they can permanently damage the reproductive tract, causing infertility for women and men.

It is very helpful for women and men to consider carefully their need for reversibility in the method they choose.

◆ How Effective Will the Method Be?

Women and men play a critical role in determining how effective a method is for them. They must understand how to use the contraceptive they choose, and they must commit themselves to using it correctly. The key to contraceptive effectiveness is consistent and correct use. Most contraceptive failures are associated with incorrect or inconsistent use. When women and men are looking for an effective and appropriate contraceptive, it is crucial to choose one that fits the reality of their lifestyles. A condom, for example, can be 97 percent effective, but only if it is used correctly every time a couple has sex.

Effectiveness rates for contraceptive methods are based on clinical studies, survey data, and scientific estimates. The U.S. Food and Drug Administration (FDA) now requires clinical studies for methods that require a prescription and for those over-the-counter methods that are developed in the future. Couples who volunteer for clinical studies report to the researchers how consistently and correctly they used the methods and whether or not they have experienced an unintended pregnancy.

Researchers use a variety of demographic and clinical data to estimate effectiveness for methods that are based on behavior and for methods whose use predates current FDA requirements for approval.

The rates of contraceptive effectiveness are measured in two ways:

- **Method-effectiveness** is the reliability of a method itself—when it is *always* used consistently and correctly. This is also called **perfect use**—the way it is intended to be used, every time.
- **Use-effectiveness** is the reliability of the method as it is *usually* used—when it is *not* always used consistently or correctly. This is also called **typical use**—the way it is used by most people.

The longer a method of contraception is used, the more effective typical use becomes. This is because typical *users* usually become more effective as they become more experienced. However, the standard measure for the effectiveness of methods is the number of unintended pregnancies experienced by every 100 women using the method during their *first* year of use.

For example, the **failure rate** of the condom with *typical use* is 14 percent. Of every 100 women whose partners use the condom, 14 will become pregnant during the first year of typical use. On the other hand, the failure rate of the condom with *perfect use* is 3 percent. Of every 100 women whose partners use the condom, only 3 will become pregnant with perfect use.

The following chart compares the typical and perfect failure rates for the methods that will be described in detail in the following chapters. It is very helpful for women and men to consider their need for effectiveness in the method they choose.

Many methods of contraception offer noncontraceptive health benefits. The male and female condoms offer protection against many STIs, including the human immunodeficiency virus (HIV), which can cause AIDS. The Pill and other hormonal methods offer health benefits ranging from menstrual regularity to protection against endometriosis, pelvic inflammatory disease (PID), and ovarian cancer. Women and men may want to consider each method's noncontraceptive health benefits as they choose the method most suited to them.

COMPARISON OF EFFECTIVENESS

Number of Pregnancies per 100 Women During First Year of Use

Method	Typical Use	Perfect Use
Continuous Abstinence	0.00	0.00
Outercourse	N/A	N/A
Norplant®	0.05	0.05
Sterilization		
Men	0.15	0.10
Women	0.5	0.5
Depo-Provera®	0.3	0.3
IUD	0.8	0.6 ParaGard® (Copper T 380A)
	2.0	1.5 Progestasert®
The Pill	5.0	0.1 combination pills
		0.5 progestin-only mini-pills
Condom	14.0	3.0
Diaphragm	20.0	6.0
Cervical Cap		
Women who have not had a child	20.0	9.0
Women who have had a child	40.0	26.0
Withdrawal	19.0	4.0
Female Condom	21.0	5.0
Periodic Abstinence	25.0	1.0 postovulation method
		2.0 symptothermal method
		3.0 cervical mucus (ovulation) method
		9.0 calendar method
Fertility Awareness Methods	N/A	N/A
Contraceptive Foam and Suppositories	26.0	6.0
Breast-Feeding	40.0	2.0-6.0 (failures occurring in first six months)
No Method	85.0	85.0

Emergency Contraception
  Emergency Contraception Pills: Treatment initiated within 72 hours of unprotected intercourse reduces the risk of pregnancy by at least 75 percent. Emergency IUD Insertion: Insertion initiated within five to seven days of unprotected intercourse reduces the risk of pregnancy by 99.9 percent.

N/A: Estimates not available

Source: Robert H. Hatcher, M.D., M.P.H., et al. *Contraceptive Technology,* 17th ed. New York: Irvington Press, 1998.

How Safe Will the Method Be?

All methods of contraception are safer than childbearing. The riskiest method is no method at all. Many methods, however, have potential side effects that can cause discomfort ranging from menstrual irregularity to headaches, nausea, and weight gain. Some methods may slightly increase the chances of certain rare, but serious, health risks, including ectopic pregnancy and stroke. Women and men should consider their ability to accept possible side effects and risks when they choose their method.

Women should consider their own medical histories and sometimes their families' medical histories when they choose contraceptive methods. Some methods are more appropriate than others for women with certain allergies or other health conditions, including diabetes, high blood pressure, heart disease, cancer of the breast or cervix, and epilepsy. Some women, or members of their families, may have a medical or physical condition that could make it dangerous or unwise to use a particular method. Each woman should consider her medical status and discuss it thoroughly with her health care professional as she chooses her contraceptive method.

Most methods are safe for nearly all women, but not in combination with some of the health risks a woman may take. Some methods, for example, are more appropriate than others for women who have more than one partner or whose partners have more than one partner. Some methods are more appropriate for women who smoke. Some are more appropriate for women who share needles for drug use or whose partners share needles for drug use. Others are more appropriate for women who go through cycles of "crash" diets. Women should weigh the impact of the health risks they take on the methods they consider.

Many women are concerned about the effect of contraception on future pregnancies. While no currently available methods are associated with the development of birth defects, some methods of contraception such as sterilization—in the rare instances in which they fail

The chart below compares the estimated annual number of deaths associated with pregnancy, abortion, and the use of various methods of birth control. With the exception of pill use by women who are heavy smokers and hysterectomy for sterilization, all methods are shown to be safer than pregnancy.

COMPARISON OF RISKS

Activity	Chance of Death in a Year
Risks for women preventing pregnancy:	
Using oral contraceptives (per year)	
Heavy Smoker	
(25 or more cigarettes per day)	1 in 1,700
Age less than 35	1 in 5,300
Age 35–44	1 in 700
Nonsmoker	1 in 66,700
Age less than 35	1 in 200,000
Age 35–44	1 in 28,000
Undergoing sterilization	
Hysterectomy	1 in 1,600
Laparoscopic tubal sterilization	1 in 38,000
Vasectomy	1 in 1,000,000
Using IUDs (per year)	1 in 10,000,000
Using diaphragm, condom, or spermicides	None
Using periodic abstinence	None
Risk per pregnancy from continuing pregnancy:	1 in 10,000
Risk from terminating pregnancy:	
Undergoing legal abortion	
Before 9 weeks	1 in 262,800
Between 9 and 12 weeks	1 in 100,000
Between 13 and 15 weeks	1 in 34,400
After 15 weeks	1 in 10,200

Source: Robert H. Hatcher, M.D., M.P.H., et al. *Contraceptive Technology,* 17th ed. New York: Irvington Press, 1998.

to prevent pregnancy—may increase the chance of ectopic pregnancy. The inappropriate use of other contraceptive methods such as the IUD may lead to infections that can cause sterility. Women should be sure to consider their future fertility as they choose their birth control method.

Will the Method Protect Against Sexually Transmitted Infections?

Only two methods of birth control—male and female condoms—offer protection against most STIs, including HIV. Spermicide may offer some protection against certain infections such as chlamydia and gonorrhea. Do not rely on any other methods to protect against STIs. Couples who choose other methods of birth control should also use male or female condoms whenever they are at risk for getting STIs. Use male or female condoms in addition to the regular method whenever:

- Either partner may have a STI.
- Either partner has more than one partner.
- Someone takes a new partner.
- Either partner shares needles to inject drugs.

How Affordable and Available Will the Method Be?

When considering the costs of protecting against unintended pregnancy, it may be helpful to consider the cost in three different ways: The short-term cost is the up-front cost—the fees that are paid to start using the method, including fees for office visits, medical exams, and the contraceptive itself. The long-term cost is the average cost over time. Other important costs to consider are the financial consequences of unintended pregnancy.

ESTIMATED COST COMPARISONS

Rough Figures Based on Surveys in 1995

Methods Listed in Order of Effectiveness—From Most to Least

Method	Short-Term, Up Front Cost (including office visit)	Cost Per Year	Five-Year Cost (including unintended pregnancies, side effects, and method)
Continuous Abstinence	$0	$0	$0
Outercourse	$0	$0	$0
Norplant®	$800	$160 (5 years)	$800
Sterilization (men)	$750	$19 (40 years)	$764
Sterilization (women)	$2,500	$63 (40 years)	$2,584
Depo-Provera®	$70	$280	$1,290
IUD	$450	$45 ParaGard® (10 years, with removal)	$540
IUD	$350	$350 Progestasert® (with removal)	$2,042
The Pill	$60	$300	$1,784
Male Condom	$6	$40 (83 acts of coitus)	$2,424
Diaphragm	$70	$130 (three years, with contraceptive jelly)	$3,666
Cervical Cap	$80	$130 (two years, with contraceptive jelly)	$5,370
Withdrawal	$0	$0	$3,278
Periodic Abstinence	$10	$0.83 (for thermometer and charts)	$3,450
Fertility Awareness Methods	$1.50	$18 (condoms for 25 acts of coitus during "unsafe" days)	N/A*
Spermicide	$12	$83 (83 acts of coitus)	$4,102
Female Condom	$2.50	$207.50 (83 acts of coitus)	$4,872
No Method	$0	$0	$14,663

* Estimates not available

Source: Robert H. Hatcher, M.D., M.P.H., et al. *Contraceptive Technology,* 17th ed. New York: Irvington Press, 1998.

While the up-front costs of certain more-effective methods may seem great, their long-term costs may compare very well with less-expensive and less-effective methods. The long-term cost of any method certainly compares well with the financial responsibilities that are associated with unintended pregnancy. The chart of cost comparisons on the opposite page compares the relative short- and long-term costs of contraceptive methods available in the United States. The figures are very rough estimates based on national averages and may not precisely reflect local costs. While actual local costs may be more or less, the chart can help women and men gauge the comparative costs of the methods they are considering. For example, costs may be less at Planned Parenthood health centers and other family planning clinics, and costs may be covered by some insurance policies. Costs for all birth control that is prescribed or indicated by a physician are reimbursable for women who are eligible for Medicaid.

Whatever method you choose, it is very important to have easy access to the method that is chosen. Some methods may be more available than others. For example, certain over-the-counter methods may be less available in your local area. Women who choose a method that requires the assistance of a health care professional must be sure that they will be able to visit their practitioners when they need to.

How Well Will a Contraceptive Method Fit into a Person's Lifestyle?

Lifestyle may be the most important factor to consider as women and men choose a contraceptive method. Methods that fit easily into a person's lifestyle are much more likely to be used effectively. Here are various questions about lifestyle that women may ask themselves in order to choose the method best suited to them:

- **How often will I have vaginal intercourse?** Women who have vaginal intercourse infrequently may decide to forego the possible side effects of the more effective hormonal prescription methods of contraception. Over-the-counter methods that are used only when sex occurs may be more appropriate for them. On the other hand, if a woman is more likely to be very anxious about using these less effective methods or if she is likely to use them inconsistently or incorrectly, the more effective hormonal methods may be more appropriate for her.

- **Am I shy about my body or embarrassed about having sex?** If so, methods that must be put in place before sex may not be appropriate.

- **Am I comfortable about having a health care professional prescribe methods for me?** Although the more effective methods of birth control are available only by prescription, some women are very uncomfortable about seeking medical assistance for contraception. They must rely on behavioral or over-the-counter methods.

- **Do I have predictable or unpredictable menstrual patterns?** Women who can predict with certainty the time of their greatest fertility may be able to choose methods that are inappropriate for women with unpredictable menstrual cycles.

- **Is uninterrupted sexual spontaneity important to me?** Women and men who find it frustrating or difficult to put barrier methods in place just before intercourse may prefer using hormonal prescription methods—or the IUD—that do not interrupt their sexual spontaneity.

- **Does my age matter?** It may. Younger people, who are more likely to have more partners and are at higher risk of STIs, will need effective protection against unintended pregnancy as well as protection against infection. Mature partners in stable and committed relationships who are building their families may be willing to use less effective methods that have fewer side effects. Older women who are approaching menopause may want more effective protection against late-in-life pregnancies. They may also want to take advantage of some of the noncontraceptive health benefits associated with hormonal methods.

- **How long do I want pregnancy prevention?** Some women and men know they want a method to work for the rest of their lives.

Some know that they want a method to work for 5 to 10 years. Others want to prevent pregnancy only for a matter of months.

- **What if I am pregnant and don't want to become pregnant again right after I have a child?** Women who plan to breast-feed a newborn must consider contraceptive methods that do not affect the quality or amount of the milk they produce.
- **How would I handle an unintended pregnancy?** Some women know that if their contraceptive method failed, they would complete the pregnancy and have a child. Others know that they would have an abortion. Women who would find it difficult to make that decision and women who would feel trapped by an unintended pregnancy may want to consider using one of the most effective methods.

How Private Does the Method Need to Be?

Many women need to keep their use of birth control as private as possible. They may have partners or family members who do not want them to use birth control. They may be living with people who would disapprove of their sexual activity, and they may fear being found out or abused. These women may prefer prescription methods, such as injections, implants, or IUDs, that cannot be discovered by people who will not honor their privacy. They may want to avoid methods that have packaging and labeling and that might be discovered in the home or purse.

To avoid embarrassment when a new method is used, women and men may want to practice using the method privately to make sure they know how to use it correctly and easily with a partner.

In the following chapters, we will look at the contraceptive options that are available to women and men in the United States. We will provide information about how these methods work, how well they work, how they are used, their advantages and disadvantages, side effects that are important to consider, and what costs are likely.

4

Reversible Contraception— Behavioral Methods

- *Continuous Abstinence*
- *Outercourse*
- *Withdrawal*
- *Periodic Abstinence or Fertility Awareness Methods (FAMs)*
- *Breast-Feeding*

Ever since the dawn of history, women and men have wanted to be able to decide when and whether to have a child. Many of the earliest methods of family planning they tried are still used by millions of women and men around the world. While these methods are most often used by people who have few alternatives, many of them are also preferred by some people who also have access to the latest advances in contraceptive technology. For thousands of years, abstinence, outercourse—sex play without intercourse—withdrawal, predicting fertility, and breast-feeding were used by our ancestors to prevent unintended pregnancy. They still play important roles in family planning today.

Continuous Abstinence

Continuous abstinence is not having vaginal intercourse. It is also called celibacy. For thousands of years, continuous abstinence has been the most effective way to avoid unintended pregnancy. Pregnancy cannot happen unless semen is deposited in the vagina or on the vulva.

Who Uses Continuous Abstinence?

All women and men abstain from vaginal intercourse at various times in their lives. About 2 percent choose to do so all their lives. Many choose to express their sexual feelings in other ways.

In American culture, most parents want their children to abstain from vaginal intercourse until they become mature enough to handle the responsibilities of sexual relationships. Many have religious beliefs that young people should abstain from vaginal intercourse until they are married.

The overwhelming social rationale for expecting kids to be abstinent is society's concern for the profound social, economic, physical, and psychological challenges that unintended pregnancy can bring to bear on a young person's life. Many young people agree that they will be better equipped to handle the risks and responsibilities of vaginal intercourse after they have become more mature. Nearly 30 percent of American teens abstain from vaginal intercourse throughout their high school years.

Adults also find that periods of continuous abstinence are sometimes appropriate for them. Many women and men remain abstinent until they establish committed relationships or during periods of illness, separation, and grief. For some women and men, the goal of abstinence from all sexual activity is an integral aspect of their contemplative or religious lifestyles.

How Well Continuous Abstinence Works

Strict and continuous abstinence from sex play between a woman and man is 100 percent effective in preventing pregnancy. It is the

Advantages of Continuous Abstinence

- Continuous abstinence from sex play is the most effective way to prevent pregnancy.
- Continuous abstinence protects against STIs, including HIV.
- Continuous abstinence has no hormonal side effects.
- Continuous abstinence does not affect a woman's natural hormonal balance.
- Many religions endorse abstinence among unmarried people.
- Continuous abstinence is immediately reversible.
- Continuous abstinence does not cost anything.

Disadvantages of Continuous Abstinence

- People may find it difficult to abstain for long periods of time.
- Women and men often end their abstinence without being prepared to protect themselves against unintended pregnancy or STIs.

only foolproof way to avoid unintended pregnancy. Pregnancy cannot happen if sperm are kept out of the vagina.

Continuous abstinence also prevents sexually transmitted infections (STIs) and is very good protection against HIV.

Outercourse

Sex play without intercourse is called outercourse. It is a way to enjoy sexual pleasure with a partner while preventing the exchange of body fluids. Preventing semen from entering the vagina protects against unintended pregnancy as well as STIs. Using techniques often regarded as foreplay, many women and men find outercourse as satisfying and pleasurable as intercourse.

A lot of people have vaginal intercourse because they think

Advantages of Outercourse

- Outercourse is the foundation for safer sex. It allows people to enjoy the pleasures of sex play without exchanging body fluids.
- Outercourse is one of the few methods that allows both partners to accept responsibility for contraception.
- Outercourse has no hormonal side effects.
- Outercourse has no barriers to interfere with physical pleasure.
- Outercourse does not affect a woman's natural hormonal balance.
- Outercourse is immediately reversible.
- Outercourse does not cost anything.
- Outercourse is always available and requires no supplies that couples can run out of or forget to use.

Outercourse also has significant advantages in its effect on sexual relationships. Partners who explore outercourse with one another may discover new sexual excitements. They may become less shy about their sexual pleasure than those who have vaginal intercourse out of a sense of obligation. Partners in outercourse may be less likely to take their sex play for granted and may be more clear about how and where they like to be caressed—they help one another enjoy sex even more. Outercourse can: improve partner communication, strengthen relationships, increase intimacy and trust, prolong sex play, enhance orgasm, add variety to sexual pleasure, and relieve anxiety.

Disadvantages of Outercourse

- People may find it difficult to abstain from vaginal intercourse for long periods of time.
- Women and men who enjoy outercourse may be tempted to have intercourse without being prepared to protect themselves against pregnancy or STIs.
- Some STIs—herpes, genital warts, and syphilis, for example—are also transmitted by skin-to-skin contact.

Outercourse—Alternatives to Intercourse

- **Masturbation.** Masturbation is the most common way we enjoy sex. Partners can enjoy it together while hugging and kissing or watching one another. Masturbating together can deepen a couple's intimacy.
- **Petting.** Kissing and fondling can be deeply pleasurable. Many partners enjoy bringing one another to orgasm with their hands.
- **Erotic massage.** Many couples enjoy arousing one another with body massage. They stimulate each other's sex organs with their hands, bodies, or mouths. They take turns bringing each other to orgasm.
- **Body rubbing** (also called frottage). Many couples rub their bodies together, especially their sex organs, for intense sexual pleasure. Many are stimulated to orgasm by this alternative to intercourse.
- **Erotica, fantasy, role play, and masks.** Reading, watching, or telling erotic fantasies with a sex partner can be exciting. Acting out fantasies can be exciting, too. Masks and costumes may intensify this kind of sex play.
- **Sex toys.** Sex toys, including vibrators and dildos, can also heighten sexual pleasure. They are used to stroke, stimulate, probe, and caress the body. Many women have learned about their capacity for orgasm while using various sex toys.

Note: If sex toys are used in foreplay or for outercourse, it's very important to keep them clean—especially if they are shared during sex play—because they can transmit STIs. Condoms can be used to cover toys that are inserted into the body. Use a fresh condom for each partner and each part of the body.

they're supposed to. For generations, women and men were taught that "good sex" meant only having an orgasm during vaginal intercourse. In fact, most women don't reach orgasm through vaginal stimulation but, instead, have orgasms when the clitoris is stimulated—whether or not they are being penetrated by a penis. Men also enjoy outercourse—even if they're shy about letting their partners know.

How Well Outercourse Works

Outercourse is nearly 100 percent effective in preventing pregnancy because fertilization of the egg cannot happen if semen is kept out of the vagina. It is possible, however, for pregnancy to result if semen is spilled on the vulva during mutual masturbation or other kinds of nonpenetrative sex play. The sperm can move through the moisture on the labia and into the vagina, then swim up into the fallopian tubes, where fertilization takes place. Couples who enjoy outercourse must be careful to keep semen away from the vulva as well as the vagina.

Outercourse helps prevent most STIs and is very good protection against HIV.

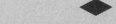

Withdrawal— "Pulling Out" (coitus interruptus)

Withdrawal is pulling the penis out of the vagina before a man ejaculates. It may be the world's oldest way to enjoy vaginal intercourse and practice birth control. It is still often used to prevent pregnancy when no other method is available, and it remains the preferred method for some couples who also have access to other methods. In the United States, withdrawal is the method of choice of about 2 percent of all couples. It is the choice of about 6 percent of sexually active unmarried women who want to prevent unintended pregnancy.

Just before a man ejaculates, he feels what physiologists call ejaculatory inevitability. This moment is a "point of no return" when ejaculation will happen—no matter what. Many men who practice withdrawal pull out of the vagina before they reach ejaculatory inevitability. Many wait until they arrive at this moment. Many others try to extend the moment for as long as possible so that they ejaculate immediately upon withdrawing.

Some men achieve orgasm and ejaculation without further stimulation after they withdraw. Others bring themselves to orgasm after withdrawing by rubbing against their partners or by masturbating. Still others postpone orgasm and ejaculation to help their partners achieve orgasm.

Advantages of Withdrawal

- Withdrawal is one of the few methods that allows a man to accept responsibility for contraception.
- Withdrawal has no hormonal side effects.
- Withdrawal has no barriers to interfere with physical pleasure.
- Withdrawal does not affect a woman's natural hormonal balance.
- Withdrawal is immediately reversible.
- Withdrawal does not cost anything and is always available.
- Withdrawal requires no supplies that couples can run out of or forget to use.

Disadvantages of Withdrawal

- Withdrawal has a relatively high failure rate.
- Pre-ejaculate can cause pregnancy.
- Not all men can be trusted to withdraw in time.
- Withdrawal offers no protection against STIs.
- Women whose partners practice withdrawal may be anxious during intercourse until their partners withdraw.
- Withdrawal may abruptly interrupt intercourse, leading to possible frustration for both partners.
- Some partners may find it messy or disagreeable for ejaculation to take place outside the vagina.

Withdrawal is effective *only* if the man pays close attention to his body's responses when he is sexually aroused. He has to understand, accept, and control the experience of ejaculatory inevitability. He must not allow the intense physical pleasure he feels at that moment to distract him from his need to withdraw. No matter how aroused he feels or how good it would feel to stay inside his partner, he must pull out to avoid ejaculating inside her vagina—even if, in the heat of passion, she urges him to stay inside her.

If a man is going to accept the couple's responsibility for preventing pregnancy, he must deeply appreciate the need to avoid pregnancy, and he must exercise great self-control. Both partners may have to sacrifice a little of their pleasure to make it work. They may, however, find other ways to enhance pleasure and orgasm after withdrawal.

How Well Withdrawal Works

Of 100 couples who practice withdrawal, about 19 of the women will become pregnant during the first year of typical use. About four will become pregnant with perfect use. One reason for these relatively high failure rates with typical use is that men dribble semen from their penises before they ejaculate. This pre ejaculate, or pre-cum, contains viable sperm that can fertilize a woman's egg. Men cannot control the oozing of pre-ejaculate, and they usually can't tell when it's happening.

Withdrawal requires great self-control, trust, and experience. It is not recommended for the sexually inexperienced and the young.

Note: Withdrawal does not protect against STIs.

Who Should Use Withdrawal?

Deciding to use withdrawal at the last minute is a lot better than nothing when no other protection is available. But the chances that withdrawal will be effective in preventing pregnancy increase if:

- The man has earned the trust of the woman and is at least as seriously concerned as she about avoiding unintended pregnancy.
- The man has experience controlling ejaculation.
- The couple tends to be less fertile than average.

Who Shouldn't Use Withdrawal?

The chances that withdrawal will fail to prevent pregnancy increase if:

- A man can't tell when he has reached ejaculatory inevitability— "the point of no return."
- The man is likely to have an early, or "premature" ejaculation— an ejaculation that occurs earlier than a man wants it to occur.
- The man is sexually inexperienced.
- The woman cannot relax and enjoy intercourse because she fears that her partner will not withdraw in time.
- The man believes it is inappropriate or unmanly to ejaculate outside the vagina.
- One partner is likely to convince the other to take a chance by not withdrawing—"just this once."

Periodic Abstinence or Fertility Awareness Methods (FAMs)

There are days when a healthy woman is fertile, days when she is infertile, and some days when fertility is unlikely but possible. In total, a woman has a good chance of becoming pregnant from unprotected vaginal intercourse over the course of about nine days of her menstrual cycle—as long as seven days before ovulation, the day of ovulation, and possibly the day after ovulation. She is less likely to become pregnant from unprotected intercourse in the day or two following ovulation, but pregnancy is possible.

A woman's fertile period depends on the life span of sperm as much as it does on the life span of her egg. The egg lives for about a day. A man's sperm can live inside a woman's body about five days, possibly seven. Recent studies show that fertilization of a woman's egg is more likely from intercourse before or during ovulation than from intercourse following ovulation. Fertilization usually occurs during a six-day period that ends in ovulation.

Understanding her monthly fertility pattern can help a woman avoid an unintended pregnancy. It can also help her plan a pregnancy. The key is for her to know when fertilization may occur by estimating the time of ovulation as nearly as possible. This must be done carefully because the timing of ovulation varies greatly from one woman to another and, for many women, from one month to the next.

A woman who monitors her fertility to prevent pregnancy may choose to abstain from vaginal intercourse for at least one-third of each menstrual cycle or to use barrier methods during that time. **Periodic abstinence** and **fertility awareness methods (FAMs)** are the two methods of contraception that depend on charting fertility patterns.

Couples who want to prevent pregnancy using periodic abstinence do not have vaginal intercourse during the woman's "unsafe days"—the days during which her fertile phase may occur. Although they abstain from vaginal intercourse during the fertile days, they may enjoy other forms of sex play.

Couples who use fertility awareness methods must use barrier contraceptives—male or female condoms, diaphragms, or cervical caps—during their fertile, or unsafe, days. They prefer to use no methods of birth control during the woman's infertile days but are willing to use barrier methods to enjoy vaginal intercourse during her fertile days.

Understanding the Menstrual Cycle

Understanding the menstrual cycle—the monthly pattern that occurs regularly in most women, from puberty to menopause—is essential for a woman's good health and is especially important if she wants to chart her fertility pattern as a method of contraception. Every menstrual cycle is divided into two parts: before ovulation and after ovulation. In a 28-day cycle, the pattern usually follows this timing:

- The beginning of the cycle, called Day 1, is the day bleeding begins. The flow usually lasts about 3 to 5 days. Usually by Day 7, certain hormones cause an egg in one ovary to start ripening. Between Days 7 and 11, the lining of the uterus begins to thicken. The influence of additional hormones after Day 11 causes the ripe egg to be released on about Day 14 in women who have a 28-day cycle. That's part one.

- In part two, the egg travels down the fallopian tube toward the uterus. If a single male sperm unites with the egg, the fertilized egg attaches to the spongy lining of the uterus. Pregnancy begins if this "implantation" occurs. If fertilization doesn't take place, the egg cell will break apart in a day or two. On about Day 25, hormone levels drop. This causes the lining of the uterus to break down, and in a few days, it is shed in a menstrual period. Another cycle has begun.

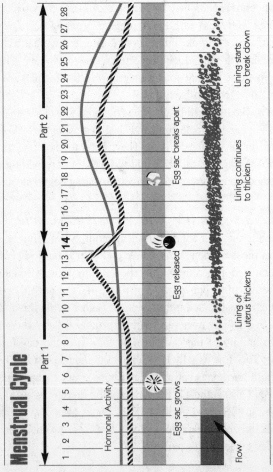

Sequence of major changes in a menstrual cycle that is 28 days long.

For some women, cycles occur fairly regularly every 28 days. But the number of days in each cycle varies from woman to woman, from every 21 to every 35 days. The first part of the cycle, from the first day of menstruation to ovulation, may vary from 13 to 20 days in length. The length of the first part is not only different from one woman to another, but is also different in many women from month to month. It is during this critical first part of the cycle that fertilization can occur. Such common circumstances as illness, physical exertion, worry, and even sudden changes in climate may occasionally upset a regular pattern by shortening it or extending it.

The second part of the cycle, from ovulation to the first day of menstruation, is about the same length in all women—the egg is released consistently 14 to 16 days before the onset of menstruation—regardless of the length of a woman's menstrual cycle.

A few women believe they can tell when the egg has been released from the ovary. Some report having a slight pain in the back or on the right or left side of the lower abdomen. This pain is sometimes referred to as *mittelschmerz*. A few may also have some increased vaginal discharge—a little blood-tinged or clear discharge from the vagina. But it is generally accepted that none of these is a *sure* signal that an egg has been released—the same symptoms can be caused by other factors.

Ways to Chart Fertility Patterns

Research conducted over the past 50 years has determined that a number of changes take place in a woman's body as part of her fertility pattern. These changes provide the signs a woman needs in order to chart her fertility. Here are brief descriptions of the methods used to chart these bodily changes in order to plan or prevent pregnancy. More complete descriptions follow.

- For the **temperature method:** Women take their body temperatures every morning before getting out of bed. Body temperature rises between 0.4°F and 0.8°F on the day of ovulation. It remains at that level until the next period.
- For the **cervical mucus method:** Women observe the changes in their cervical mucus. They do so all through the first part of the

menstrual cycle, until ovulation has occurred. Normally cloudy, tacky mucus will become clear and slippery in the few days before ovulation. It also will stretch between the fingers. This happens at the most fertile phase. To prevent pregnancy during this time, couples abstain from vaginal intercourse or use barrier contraceptives (male or female condoms, diaphragms, or cervical caps). The cervical mucus method is sometimes called the **ovulation** or **Billings method.**

- For the **calendar,** or **"rhythm,"** method: Women chart menstrual cycles on calendars. Ovulation may be predicted if periods are the same every month. Couples abstain or use a barrier contraceptive during the unsafe days. It will be more difficult to predict the day of ovulation if cycle length varies from month to month. In that case, there will be more unsafe days. (It is best not to rely on this method alone.)

    The temperature method, the cervical mucus method, and the calendar method work best in combination with each other. This combination is called the **symptothermal method.**

- Couples also combine these charting methods for the **postovulation method** of contraception. They abstain from vaginal intercourse or use withdrawal or a barrier method from the beginning of the woman's period until the morning of the fourth day after her predicted ovulation. A woman is much less likely to be fertile after ovulation has occurred (postovulation). However, couples who practice the postovulation method must abstain from vaginal intercourse or use withdrawal for a barrier method for more than half of the woman's menstrual cycle.

How Well These Methods Work for Contraception

Of 100 couples who use any of these methods for one year, 25 women will become pregnant with typical use. The failure rate is higher for single women. Combining the various methods with careful and consistent use and having no unprotected vaginal intercourse during the fertile phase can give better results.

Of 100 couples who use the **postovulation method** for one year with perfect use, only one woman will become pregnant.

Of 100 couples who use the **symptothermal method** for one year with perfect use, two women will become pregnant.

Of 100 couples who use the **cervical mucus method** for one year with perfect use, three women will become pregnant.

Of 100 couples who use the **calendar method** for one year with perfect use, nine women will become pregnant.

These methods require keeping consistent and accurate records. Some skill is required in calculating, and the margin for error depends on how accurately signs and records are interpreted and followed. It is most important that original explanations, early coaching, and frequent follow-up be done by a professional instructor or successful users. These methods work better for women whose cycles are regular and of the same length.

Women who are breast-feeding or approaching menopause may find it more difficult to chart their fertility patterns. Their fertile signs may vary in unpredictable ways due to irregular hormonal fluctuations. Likewise, multiorgasmic women are also likely to ovulate unpredictably.

If a woman is using the Pill and is planning to switch to periodic abstinence, she must stop taking the Pill and use another method of contraception, such as a barrier method (male or female condoms, diaphragms, or cervical caps), while learning the ways to predict her fertility pattern. Hormones in the Pill alter the natural menstruation and fertility cycle.

A woman should not depend on predicting fertility if:

- She has irregular periods.
- Her partner is unwilling to observe periods of abstinence from vaginal intercourse or use barrier methods at fertile times.
- She has an STI or frequent abnormal vaginal discharge.
- She cannot keep careful records.

Charting fertility patterns requires dedication, education, and practice. It is most effective when both partners are mature, responsible, and committed to making them work. That's why it is very important for both partners to learn the fundamentals and support each other in observing the abstinence or contraceptive use that is required.

Now, let's take a closer look at the methods to chart fertility patterns.

Temperature Method

One of the changes that ordinarily take place in a woman's body as part of her menstrual pattern is that her body temperature is lower during the first part of the cycle. In most women, it usually rises slightly with ovulation and remains up during the second part until just before her next period. Recording each day's temperature helps to indicate when ovulation has occurred.

The temperature method requires that a woman chart her basal body temperature (BBT), the temperature the body registers when completely at rest. BBT varies slightly from person to person. For most women, a temperature of 96° to 98°F, recorded orally, is considered normal before ovulation and 97° to 99°F after ovulation. The changes are small fractions—from one-tenth to one-half degree. The best thermometer to use is a special large-scale, easy-to-read one that registers only from 96° to 100°F. A rectal or oral basal temperature thermometer can be bought in most drugstores for about $10. Generally, rectal readings are more reliable, but whichever she uses, a woman should take her temperature the same way every day.

TAKING BASAL BODY TEMPERATURE

A woman must measure body temperature before getting out of bed, talking, eating, drinking, having sex, or smoking. She should insert the thermometer in the rectum or the mouth for a full five minutes, if it is not a battery-operated thermometer. The temperature should be read to within one-tenth of a degree and recorded.

Simple morning activities—such as getting out of bed, urinating, eating, drinking water, or even speaking—may cause the body's temperature to rise. That's why it's very important to take the BBT immediately upon awakening—before getting out of bed. Illness, emotional distress, jet lag, disturbed sleep, smoking, drinking an unaccustomed amount of alcohol the night before, and using an electric blanket may also affect BBT. It is likely to be one-tenth of a degree higher for each hour that one sleeps later than usual.

Such disturbances of BBT should be noted in a special place provided on the BBT chart. It will be helpful to recognize fluctuations that occurred because "baby woke me, 6 a.m.," "drank half a bottle of wine last night," or "feeling stressed about mom." Occasional disturbances needn't jeopardize the ability to use BBT to prevent pregnancy.

Because it's important to take BBT before any activity whatsoever, it's a good idea to prepare everything the night before. The thermometer should be shaken down to 96°F and placed within easy reach (not near a hot place), and the bulb lubricated if it's going to be used rectally.

Not every woman charts her fertility patterns first thing in the morning. Some do so at specially set times during the day or evening. To establish basal body temperature, they rest and don't eat or drink anything for an hour before taking their temperature.

CHARTING THE TEMPERATURE PATTERN

Each reading must be recorded. Charts for this purpose may be obtained from a doctor or family planning clinic, or photocopies can be made of the sample chart on page 66. As each day's temperature is plotted on the graph, the pattern will become clear. The temperature rise may be sudden, gradual, or in steps. The nature of the pattern may even vary from menstrual cycle to menstrual cycle. BBT can be influenced by physical or emotional upsets or even lack of sleep. Noting such events on the chart helps to interpret the readings.

In the beginning, a woman can get help in reading the BBT chart from a physician, nurse, or family planning specialist. Knowledge and confidence to use the chart without supervision will be gained after a while.

Note: A woman must be sure to chart her temperature for at least three months before relying on this method.

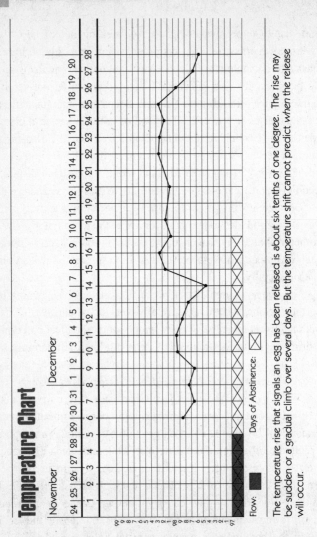

Temperature Chart

The temperature rise that signals an egg has been released is about six tenths of one degree. The rise may be sudden or a gradual climb over several days. But the temperature shift cannot predict *when* the release will occur.

DETERMINING THE SAFE TIMES

After the temperature rise has lasted for at least three days, the safe days have begun. They will last until the temperature drop that usually comes just before the onset of the next menstrual period. For complete protection, a woman should consider unsafe all the days between the start of the period and start of the fourth day of the next temperature rise. Such caution is necessary because the temperature method is quite accurate at detecting when ovulation has occurred, but it cannot predict when it's *about to* happen. The other important reason that the entire first part of the cycle must be considered unsafe has to do with the life expectancy of a man's sperm. Sperm generally remain capable of fertilizing an egg for two to three days after ejaculation. There are even rare instances of sperm remaining active five or more days after intercourse.

If vaginal intercourse occurs several days before ovulation, there is a good chance that live sperm could still fertilize a newly released egg. If a woman combines BBT with another charting method, she may be able to calculate ovulation in advance.

Women who become confident about using their BBT to determine their safe days may not need to take their temperatures between the start of the infertile time and the beginning of their next menstrual periods.

Cervical Mucus Method

The cervical mucus method is based on another change that occurs during the menstrual cycle. The hormones that control menstrual cycle phases also act on the glands of the cervix that produce mucus secretions. The mucus secreted by the cervix collects on the cervix and in the vagina. It changes in quality and quantity just before and during ovulation. With proper personal instruction, many women can learn to recognize the changing characteristics. Instruction in the cervical mucus method is usually given on a one-to-one basis.

RECOGNIZING THE MUCUS PATTERN

- The cycle begins with menstruation. During vaginal bleeding, the flow disguises the mucus signs.
- The menstrual period is usually followed by a few days when no mucus is present. These are "dry days."
- As an egg starts to ripen, mucus increases in the vagina and appears at the vaginal opening. It is generally yellow or white, cloudy, and sticky.
- The greatest amount of cervical mucus during the "wet days" usually occurs immediately before ovulation during the "slip-

Mucus Pattern

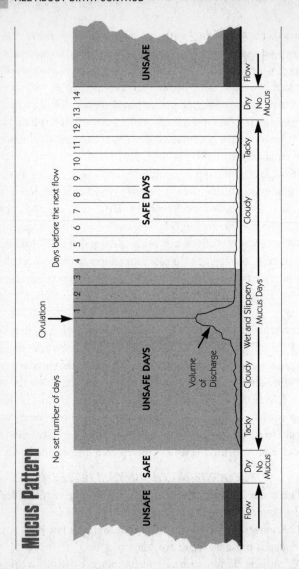

pery days." The mucus takes on a clear and slippery quality that resembles raw egg whites. When the mucus can be stretched between the fingers, it is called **spinnbarkeit**—German for "stretchability." This is the peak period of fertility.

- About four days after the wet days begin, mucus may abruptly become cloudy and sticky, then reduce sharply in volume, and a few dry days may return before menstruation begins.

CHARTING THE MUCUS PATTERN

As with the other methods, records need to be kept. It's suggested that a woman chart her observation daily on a calendar. She should mark the days of the menstrual period, the dry days, the wet days, and the

Charting Your Mucus Pattern
August

Sunday	Monday	Tuesday	Wednesday	Thursday	Friday	Saturday
		Tacky 1	Dry 2	Dry 3	Dry 4	Flow 5
Flow 6	Flow 7	Flow 8	Dry 9	Dry 10	Tacky 11 (white)	Tacky 12
Tacky 13	Tacky 14 (more)	Tacky 15	Wet 16	Slippery 17 Ovulation	Slippery 18 Ovulation	Slippery 19
Tacky 20	Tacky 21	Dry 22	Dry 23	Dry 24	Tacky 25	Dry 26
Dry 27	Dry 28	Dry 29	Dry 30	Flow 31		

slippery days. It's best for a woman to avoid intercourse for at least one whole cycle when she starts to use the mucus method for birth control. She should get someone with experience to help her become familiar with her own pattern until she is able to interpret the changes herself.

A woman can check her mucus in several ways, depending on which is most comfortable for her. She can:

- wipe the vaginal opening with toilet tissue before urination
- observe the discharge on underpants
- obtain some of the mucus by placing her fingers (making sure they are clean) in the vagina

She should check several times a day when there is any sign of mucus.

This method is less reliable for women who produce little mucus or if the natural mucus pattern is altered by:

- using douches, "feminine hygiene" products, or contraceptive foams, creams, jellies, or suppositories
- surgery that is performed on the cervix—especially if cryotherapy or a loop electrosurgical excision procedure is used
- vaginitis
- STIs
- breast-feeding
- perimenopause
- recent use of hormonal contraceptives

Women who ovulate on Day 7 or 8 may produce too little mucus to use this method.

DETERMINING THE SAFE TIMES

- It is considered unsafe to have vaginal intercourse during menstruation, especially during shorter cycles, because vaginal bleeding disguises the mucus signs.
- Nonmenstrual vaginal bleeding around the time of ovulation may be mistaken for a menstrual period.
- Intercourse may, however, take place during the brief period of safe dry days that may follow menstruation in a long cycle.

- The fertile phase begins at the first sign of wetness after menstruation, but it may also begin a day or two before wetness appears. Intercourse must be avoided on any wet day, unless pregnancy is desired—fertilization is most likely to occur during this phase. A woman who does not want to become pregnant must refrain from vaginal intercourse for at least three days after ovulation or until the wet days end, whichever is the longer number of days.
- It is considered safe to have sex after ovulation when mucus sharply decreases in volume and becomes cloudy and sticky again. It is considered even safer to have intercourse during the dry days that may follow before menstruation begins.

Note: Fewer pregnancies occur when intercourse takes place only on the dry days.

Calendar Method

The calendar method attempts to predict ovulation using a woman's menstrual history. A written record is kept—an ordinary calendar can be used to note each cycle, counting from the first day of one menstrual period up to, but not including, the first day of the next. The day bleeding starts is Day 1, and this is marked by circling that date on the calendar. Continue to circle Day 1 for at least 8 months (12 is better). Then count the days in each cycle.

Of course, there is no assurance that cycle variations will remain the same. So a woman must continue to circle each Day 1 and list the length of her last cycle.

KNOWING THE ROLE
OF THE CALENDAR METHOD

These rules can help a woman find out only a couple of days in advance when she *probably* will ovulate. Calendar records should *only* be used with the other charting methods that have been explained. Using all of them together is called the **symptothermal method.** A general rule is to always be guided by any sign of fertility. The calendar method is especially chancy if a woman's cycles are not always the same length.

CHARTING THE MENSTRUAL PATTERN

The woman keeps a record of the number of days in each cycle. When bleeding starts, she circles the date on the calendar.

To find the first day of likely infertility, a woman should check the record of previous months and find the shortest cycle, then subtract 18

Cycle Record

First Day of Period	Number of Days in Preceding Cycle	First Day of Period	Number of Days in Preceding Cycle
Jan. 20	29	May 12	26
Feb. 18	29	June 9	28
Mar. 18	28	July 9	30
Apr. 16	29	Aug. 5	27

from the total number of days in that cycle. For example, if the short-est cycle is 26 days long, she'd subtract 18 from 26, which leaves 8. Starting with the circled date (the first day of the current cycle), she would count ahead eight days and draw an X through that second date. That's the first day of likely fertility and, therefore, the first day of abstinence or contraceptive use. But if the BBT chart shows even a slight shift before that, the couple shouldn't have unprotected vaginal intercourse until three full days after the temperature rise.

The Safe Times (Calendar Method)

Sunday	Monday	Tuesday	Wednesday	Thursday	Friday	Saturday
Safe Day (1) Start of Period	Safe Day 2	Safe Day 3	Safe Day 4	Safe Day 5	Safe Day 6	Safe Day 7)
8 (X)	9	10	11	12	13	14
15	16	17	18	19 (X)	Safe Day (20	Safe Day 21
Safe Day 22	Safe Day 23	Safe Day 24	Safe Day 25	Safe Day 26	Safe Day 27	Safe Day 28
Safe Day 29	Safe Day 30)					

Start of Period: ◯   Safe Days: ( )

To find the last day of abstinence or contraceptive use with the calendar method, the woman subtracts 11 days from the longest cycle. For example, if the longest cycle is 30 days, then 30 minus 11 is 19. Starting from the first circle, she should count 19 days and draw an X through that date also. Cycles should be charted for at least three to six months before the safe days are calculated. Other methods should be used to confirm the calculations.

DETERMINING THE SAFE TIMES

Safe times are likely from the first day of menstruation, Day 1, which is circled, to the first X (Days 1 through 7 in the example). They are also likely from the second X to the next circle (Days 20 through 30 in the example). Unsafe days appear between the two Xs.

Remember: If all the cycles are shorter than 27 days, a woman shouldn't try to use calendar estimates at all. The first part of any cycle may be irregular. Trying to add a few days of vaginal intercourse in the early part of the cycle can be risky when attempting to prevent an unplanned pregnancy. Learning the meaning of changes in the normal vaginal discharge may reduce miscalculations. But a woman should always be guided by any of the symptothermal signs of fertility.

Symptothermal Method

Using all three fertility awareness methods—temperature, cervical mucus, and calendar—is called the symptothermal method. The symptothermal method allows a woman to be more accurate in predicting her safe days than if she uses any one of the methods alone. When she is using these methods together, the signs of one can serve to confirm those of the other. For example, a record of the mucus pattern can be useful because elevated temperature resulting from illness or emotional stress may be confusing. Combining methods also permits vaginal intercourse during the early dry days and shortens the period of abstinence that is necessary for complete protection when using the temperature method alone.

Products to Use with These Methods

At this time no device has been approved by the U.S. Food and Drug Administration that can simplify or ensure greater success with any of these methods. From time to time, announcements are made of patented items to help in calendar calculation or to test mucus change by chemically treated paper or of other products under development for this purpose. None has proven any more reliable for strictly contraceptive purposes. Success in the use of any of these methods for predicting fertility is the result of good initial instruction, persistence, accuracy in keeping records, and cooperation by both partners in the discipline involved.

Test kits that attempt to predict ovulation are available for home use. They may be useful for planning pregnancies but are not reliable for purposes of birth control. Sperm can live in the fallopian tubes up to seven days. So pregnancy often results from having unprotected vaginal intercourse during the six days before ovulation.

Who Should Use Periodic Abstinence or FAMs?

If a woman's lifestyle makes it difficult for her to consistently chart her fertility and abstain or use barrier methods during unsafe days, these finely tuned methods will probably not work for her. For example, if a woman and her partner are away from one another a good deal, periodic abstinence and FAMs may be very difficult to maintain. The chances are that they may be apart on safe days and together on unsafe days. The times they could have vaginal intercourse safely might become very limited, and they may become very tempted to take risks.

Charting the woman's fertility pattern may work if:

- The woman has received careful instruction in the methods.
- The woman has only one sex partner and he is equally committed to the methods she wants to use.
- The woman has the self-discipline required to check and chart her fertility signs and observe the rules.
- The couple doesn't mind abstaining or using withdrawal or barrier methods for the first part of the cycle.

Charting the woman's fertility pattern may not work if:
- The woman has more than one sex partner.
- The woman's sex partner isn't equally committed to the methods she wants to use.
- The woman is temperamentally unsuited for keeping close track of her fertile days.
- The woman or man has doubts about being able to abstain from vaginal intercourse or using a barrier method for about 10 days each month.
- The woman wouldn't consider having an abortion although she has a medical condition that poses a grave danger for her if she were to become pregnant.
- The woman is taking medication that may affect her cervical mucus, body temperature, or menstrual regularity.

Cost

Some couples chart the woman's fertility pattern to prevent pregnancy because it is economical, safe, and can be discontinued easily when pregnancy is desired. Little equipment is needed, and calendars, thermometers, and charts are widely available. No medication is involved, which is especially appealing to women who have physical or health conditions that might make other forms of birth control less desirable or unsuitable. Medical checkups are not required for these methods, although professional instruction is important. Also, periodic abstinence is acceptable to most religions.

Charts for graphing fertility signs and patterns cost little or nothing. They are available at family planning clinics and from private instructors and organizations. Basal body temperature thermometers cost about $10.

It may be necessary to pay a fee for classes to learn fertility awareness techniques. It is very helpful if both partners attend the sessions so that each will be aware of precisely how these methods work. Fertility awareness methods require dedication, education, and

Comparison of Duration of Periods of Abstinence

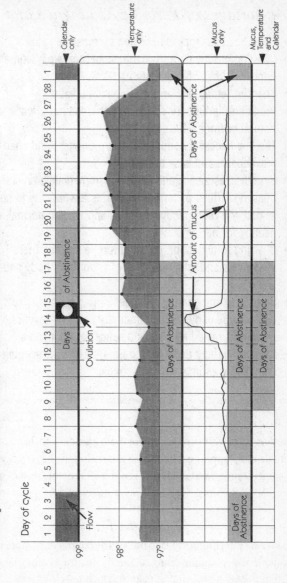

Advantages of Periodic Abstinence and FAMs:

- Periodic abstinence is accepted by most religions.
- Charting fertility patterns can be used to help a woman conceive when she is ready.
- Charting fertility patterns has no side effects.
- Predicting fertility for contraception does not affect a woman's natural hormonal balance.
- The few necessary supplies—thermometers and charts—are inexpensive and easy to find.
- Periodic abstinence and FAMs are immediately reversible.
- Charting fertility patterns familiarizes a woman with her sexual and reproductive systems and what is normal and healthy for her.
- Charting fertility patterns can improve both partners' awareness and understanding of a woman's body and how it works.
- Observing and charting changes during the menstrual cycle can provide early clues to infertility or other sexual health problems, including STIs and cancer of the cervix.
- Charting fertility patterns and the mutual contraceptive effort can deepen intimacy for the couple.

practice. It is very important for both partners to learn the fundamentals and support each other in observing the abstinence required. In some states, Medicaid will cover the cost of classes taken at a clinic or when authorized by a private physician.

Finding a Teacher

Classes on charting fertility patterns for contraception are offered by many family planning clinics, family health centers, and church-affiliated instructors, and at Catholic hospitals.

Instruction in a religious setting may reflect the tenets of that

- Charting fertility patterns can help a woman with premenstrual syndrome become more aware of the timing of her symptoms so that she can seek solutions.

Disadvantages of Periodic Abstinence and FAMs:

- Periodic abstinence and FAMs are very "unforgiving"; intercourse one time on a fertile day can lead to a pregnancy. The typical use failure rate is higher than that of most other methods.
- Periodic abstinence requires that the woman and man abstain from vaginal intercourse from 10 to 16 days each month.
- Periodic abstinence and FAMs provide no protection against STIs.
- Periodic abstinence and FAMs require a high level of motivation, long-term commitment, and the cooperation of both partners.
- Periodic abstinence and FAMs take much longer to learn to use than other contraceptive methods do.
- Periodic abstinence and FAMs call for more continuous discipline and self-control than other contraceptive methods do.

religion. For nonsectarian instruction, a woman may ask for a referral from a Planned Parenthood health center, a women's clinic that is not affiliated with a religious group, or a state or county health department.

An information packet that includes a basic overview, a book list, addresses of resource organizations, and information on how to find a teacher is available for $4 and a self-addressed, stamped business envelope from the Fertility Awareness Network, P.O. Box 2606, New York, NY 10009. For Catholic-based instruction, contact a Catholic hospital or the offices of the local archdiocese.

Fertility Pattern Chart

Month/Day																																				
Cycle Day	1	2	3	4	5	6	7	8	9	10	11	12	13	14	15	16	17	18	19	20	21	22	23	24	25	26	27	28	29	30	31	32	33	34	35	36	37

Temperature

- 99°
- 98.8
- 98.6
- 98.4
- 98.2
- 98°
- 97.8
- 97.6
- 97.4
- 97.2
- 97°

MUCUS Wet, Dry, Cloudy, Clear, Tacky, etc.																																				
Notes																																				
Intercourse																																				

When deciding which group to approach, a woman should keep in mind that religion-oriented groups that teach "natural family planning" are likely to encourage only periodic abstinence. They may discourage the use of barrier methods with fertility awareness. Organizations that teach "fertility awareness methods" are more likely to teach the optional use of barrier methods.

Breast-Feeding—Lactational Amenorrhea Method (LAM)

Breast-feeding prevents ovulation and causes temporary infertility. The stimulation of the nipples encourages the production of prolactin, a hormone necessary for the production of breast milk. It also inhibits the secretion of gonadotropin, a hormone necessary for ovulation. Without the release of an egg, pregnancy cannot take place.

Breast-feeding as birth control is called the **lactational amenorrhea method (LAM).** LAM can be effective for six months after delivery only if a woman:

- has not had a period since she delivered her baby
- suckles her baby at least six times a day on both breasts
- suckles her baby "on demand" at least every four hours during the day
- provides nighttime breast-feedings at least every six hours—does not let her baby sleep through the night
- does not substitute other foods for a breast-milk meal
- does not rely on the method after six months

Supplemental feedings become essential for the good health of the baby after six months. The reduction in breast-feeding stimulates the return of ovulation.

Women who work outside the home can rely on LAM by pumping their milk at work or elsewhere during the day. Pumping every four hours stimulates the nipples enough to control the flow of the necessary hormones. The milk can be refrigerated or frozen and bottle-fed to the baby in the mother's absence.

Safe and effective contraceptives for breast-feeding mothers include:

- barrier methods—male and female condoms, diaphragm, or cervical cap
- progestin-only hormonal methods—mini-pills, Norplant, Depo-Provera. (The combination birth control pill is not a good option for breast-feeding mothers because it contains estrogen, which decreases the production of milk.)
- IUDs

How Well LAM Works

Out of 100 women who use LAM, two to six will become pregnant with perfect use in the first six months. Up to 40 will become pregnant with typical use in the first six months.

Some women who rely on LAM incorrectly believe that they will not ovulate until after their first period. It is important to remember that ovulation occurs *before* menstruation. If a woman relying on LAM has a period, even a very light one, she should consult her health care provider immediately and use another method of birth control.

LAM does not offer protection against STIs.

LAM is more successful for women in the developing world. The reasons may be that:

- Nursing women in developing countries are less likely to have sexual intercourse. Many of their cultures frown on men having sex with nursing mothers.
- The return of ovulation is associated with nutrition and well being.
- Nursing women in developing countries often carry their infants with them most of the day, increasing the likelihood of feeding on demand.

Advantages of LAM

Breast-feeding has many health advantages for the baby.
• Breast-feeding provides the best nutrition.
• Breast-feeding passes on some of the mother's antibodies to protect the baby from certain bacteria and viruses.
• Breast-feeding decreases the likelihood of infection from germs in water, other milk, or formula.
• Breast-feeding increases body contact and enhances comfort for the child and bonding between mother and child.
• Breast-feeding protects against the development of allergies and may protect against the development of asthma.

LAM also has advantages for mothers.
• LAM is effective for up to six months after delivery.
• LAM is inexpensive.
• LAM is immediately effective.
• LAM reduces bleeding after delivery.
• LAM requires no supplies or medical supervision. Women may initially benefit from consulting with a lactation expert, and they should be assisted as soon as possible if problems arise so that lactation is not disrupted.
• LAM does not affect a woman's natural hormonal balance.

Disadvantages of LAM

• LAM must be used correctly and consistently, or else there are very high failure rates.
• LAM can be relied on for only six months.
• LAM does not protect against STIs.
• Breast-feeding on demand may be difficult given many women's lifestyles.

For more information on breast-feeding, contact:

American Academy of Pediatrics
141 Northwest Point Blvd.
P.O. Box 927
Elk Grove, IL 60009-0927
847-981-7945
http:\\www.aap.org

La Leche League International
1400 N. Meacham Rd.
P.O. Box 4079
Schaumburg, IL 60168
800-LA-LECHE
847-519-7730
http://www.prairienet.org/llli/

- *Condom*
- *Female Condom*
- *Lubricants*
- *Contraceptive Foams, Creams, Jellies, and Suppositories*
- *Diaphragm and Cervical Cap*
- *Latex Allergy*

Barrier methods of contraception prevent the sperm from entering the uterus and swimming up the fallopian tubes to join with the egg.

Diaphragms and cervical caps and the spermicides in contraceptive foams, creams, jellies, and suppositories were invented to prevent pregnancy. The condom—one of the world's oldest and most popular methods of contraception—was originally devised to protect the wearer from sexually transmitted infections (STIs). The newer female condom is designed to do both. All these methods are immediately effective and immediately reversible.

The barriers provided by the male and female condom, diaphragm, and cap are membranes that block sperm from entering the uterus. Spermicides are chemicals that weaken sperm and block their movement.

As with all barrier methods, practice makes perfect. Women and men who decide to use a barrier method for the first time can improve effectiveness if they practice inserting it or putting it on before using it with a sex partner.

Condom

A condom is a sheath made of latex, plastic, or animal tissue that fits over the penis. Also called a rubber, safe, or jimmy, a condom catches semen before, during, and after a man ejaculates. Condoms protect against unintended pregnancy by keeping sperm out of the vagina.

They also offer protection for both partners against STIs by preventing the exchange of infected body fluids during vaginal, anal, and oral intercourse.

How Well Condoms Work in Preventing Pregnancy

Of 100 women whose partners use condoms, about 14 will become pregnant during the first year of typical use. Three will become pregnant with perfect use.

Protection against unintended pregnancy is increased if contraceptive foams, creams, jellies, or suppositories are used along with the condom. These contain spermicides and can immobilize sperm if the condom breaks. Some condoms are coated with a spermicide such as nonoxynol-9, which is used in many vaginal contraceptives to increase effectiveness in preventing pregnancy.

Latex condoms protect against many sexually transmitted infections, including HIV, the human immunodeficiency virus that can cause AIDS. In fact, latex condoms offer better protection against STIs than any other birth control method—except continuous abstinence.

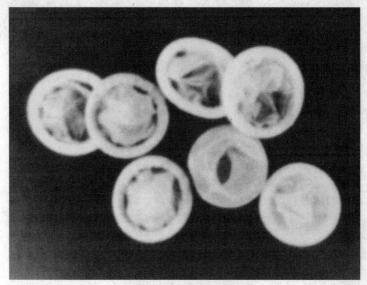

MALE CONDOMS

Latex condoms offer good protection against:
- vaginitis caused by infections like trichomoniasis
- pelvic inflammatory disease (PID), which can cause sterility
- gonorrhea
- chlamydia
- syphilis
- chancroid
- human immunodeficiency virus (HIV)

Latex condoms offer some protection against:
- human papilloma virus (HPV), which can cause genital warts
- herpes simplex virus (HSV), which can cause genital herpes
- hepatitis-B virus

Latex condoms may even reduce a woman's chance of getting cervical cancer. They offer some protection against the kinds of HPV infections associated with cervical cancer.

Condoms and Protection against HIV

Condoms have a very good record of protecting against the transmission of HIV. In a 1987–1991 study of couples in which one partner had HIV, all 123 couples who used condoms every time they had sexual intercourse for four years prevented the transmission of HIV. In 122 couples who did not use condoms every time, 12 partners became infected.

A similar 1993 study showed that using condoms every time prevented HIV transmission for all but 2 of 171 women who had male partners with HIV. However, 8 out of 10 women whose partners didn't use condoms every time became infected.

Condoms made from animal tissue or plastic are not recommended for protection against STIs. Some viruses, such as hepatitis-B and HIV, may be small enough to pass through the pores of the animal tissue, and plastic condoms have not undergone enough testing to be *proven* effective. However, use of these condoms still protects better against STIs than no protection at all.

The Pill, IUD, Depo-Provera, vasectomy, and tubal sterilization offer greater protection against pregnancy than condoms but no protection against STIs. Many people use latex condoms along with these and other methods for the best protection against both pregnancy and STIs.

How to Use Condoms

Handle condoms gently. Store them in a cool, dry place. Long exposure to air, heat, and light makes them more breakable. Do not stash them continually in a back pocket, wallet, or glove compartment.

Use lubricant inside and outside the condom. (Many condoms are prelubricated.) Lubrication helps prevent rips and tears and increases sensitivity. Use only water-based lubricants, such as K-Y® lubricating jelly, with latex condoms. Oil-based lubricants, such as

For increased effectiveness against pregnancy and STIs:

- The man should pull out immediately if he feels the condom breaking or falling off.
- A fresh condom should be used for each act of intercourse.
- A fresh condom should be used if partners switch from anal to vaginal intercourse.
- A fresh condom should be used on sex toys for each different partner and for each part of the body.
- Partners should keep an adequate supply of condoms on hand for repeated intercourse, replacement of broken condoms, or when sex play is interrupted and resumed.

petroleum jelly, cold cream, butter, and mineral and vegetable oils, damage latex.

PUTTING ON A CONDOM

For pleasure, ease, and effectiveness, both partners should know how to put on and use a condom. To learn without feeling pressured or embarrassed, practice on your penis or a penis-shaped object such as a ketchup bottle, banana, cucumber, or squash. Remember: Practice makes perfect.

Put the condom on before the penis touches the vulva. Men leak fluids from their penises before and after ejaculation. Pre-ejaculate can carry enough sperm to cause pregnancy. It can also carry enough germs to cause STIs.

Use a condom only once. Use a fresh one for each erection. Always have a good supply on hand.

Condoms usually come rolled into a ring shape. They are individually sealed in aluminum foil or plastic. Be careful—don't tear the condom while unwrapping it. If it is brittle, stiff, or sticky, throw it away and use another.

PUTTING ON A CONDOM

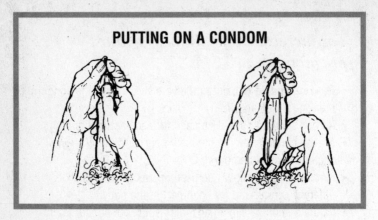

- Put a drop or two of lubricant inside the rolled condom.
- Place the rolled condom over the tip of the hard penis.
- Leave a half-inch space at the tip to collect semen.
- If the penis is not circumcised, pull back the foreskin before rolling on the condom.
- Pinch the air out of the tip with one hand. (Friction against air bubbles causes most condom breaks.)
- Unroll the condom over the penis with the other hand.
- Roll it all the way down to the base of the penis.
- Smooth out any air bubbles.
- Lubricate the outside of the condom.

TAKING OFF A CONDOM
- Pull out before the penis softens.
- Don't spill the semen. Hold the condom against the base of the penis while it is pulled out.
- Throw the condom away.
- Wash the penis with soap and water before embracing again.

IF A CONDOM BREAKS...
If a condom breaks *during* intercourse, the man should pull out quickly and replace the broken condom with a new one. Men should be able to tell if a condom breaks during intercourse. To learn what it feels like, they can break condoms on purpose while masturbating.

Any semen that leaks out should be washed away with soap and water. If semen leaks into the vagina during a woman's fertile period, there is a possibility pregnancy may occur. A woman may want to contact her clinician to discuss this.

All condoms are tested for defects. Each latex condom is formed on a hollow glass mold that is shaped like a penis. A mild electric current is used to test each condom. If the current passes through the condom, the condom is defective. A stream of air blows defective condoms off onto the factory floor, where they are swept up and recycled. Thousands of them are shredded and used to stuff the upholstery in automobiles.

Like rubber bands, latex condoms deteriorate with age. The expiration date or date of manufacture is printed on the wrapper of each condom. If properly stored, a condom may be used until the expiration date or five years after the date of manufacture. If a condom is brittle, stiff, or sticky, ignore the date on the wrapper and throw it away—it has deteriorated and will not protect you or your partner.

Side Effects

Condoms have no side effects except for people who are allergic to latex (see page 111). Five to 7 percent of women and men have such

(continued on page 80)

A Condom by Any Other Name...

Condoms work, no matter what you or your partner call them—and they are called by a lot of names. Here are just a few of the more colorful ones: rubber • nightcap • raincoat • protection • jimmy hat • diving suit • buckskin • French tickler • French letter • English letter • American letter • Italian letter • Spanish letter • Greek cap • Manhattan eel • Coney Island whitefish • jo-bag • kinga • manhole cover • safe • rubber duckie.

Don't Let Embarrassment Become a Health Risk

If you are embarrassed to talk with your partner about using condoms, practice before you are in a sexual situation. Then choose the right time to talk—don't wait until the heat of passion takes over. It may overwhelm your good intentions.

Don't be shy—be direct. Be honest about your feelings and needs. Talking with your partner about using condoms makes it easier for you both. It can help create a relaxed mood to make sex more enjoyable. While it may be difficult to talk about using condoms, it will be easier if you are in a loving relationship that makes you feel happy and good about yourself and your partner. In any case, don't let embarrassment become a health risk. The following script may give you some ideas.

If Your Partner Says: What's that?
You Can Say: A condom, sweetheart.
If Your Partner Says: What for?
You Can Say: To use when we're making love.
If Your Partner Says: I don't like using them.
You Can Say: Why not?
If Your Partner Says: It doesn't feel as good with a rubber.
You Can Say: I'll feel more relaxed. If I'm more relaxed, I can make it feel better for you.
If Your Partner Says: But we've never used a condom before.
You Can Say: I don't want to take any more risks.
If Your Partner Says: Rubbers are gross.
You Can Say: Being pregnant when I don't want to be is more gross. Getting AIDS is totally gross.
If Your Partner Says: Don't you trust me?
You Can Say: Trust isn't the point. People carry STIs without knowing it.
If Your Partner Says: I'll pull out in time.
You Can Say: Women can get pregnant from pre-ejaculate. You can get STIs from pre-ejaculate, too.
If Your Partner Says: I thought you said using condoms made you feel cheap.

You Can Say: I decided to face facts. I like having sex and I want to stay healthy and happy.

If Your Partner Says: Rubbers aren't romantic.

You Can Say: What's more romantic than making love and protecting each other's health at the same time?

If Your Partner Says: Let's face it. Making love with a rubber on is like taking a shower with a raincoat on.

You Can Say: You face it. Doing it without a rubber isn't making love—it's playing Russian roulette.

If Your Partner Says: It just isn't as sensitive.

You Can Say: Maybe that way it will last even longer and that will make up for it.

If Your Partner Says: I don't stay hard when I put on a condom.

You Can Say: I can do something about that.

If Your Partner Says: Putting it on interrupts everything.

You Can Say: Not if we both help put it on.

If Your Partner Says: I'll try, but it might not work.

You Can Say: Practice makes perfect.

If Your Partner Says: But I love you.

You Can Say: Then you'll help me protect myself.

If Your Partner Says: I guess you don't really love me.

You Can Say: I do, but I'm not risking my future to prove it.

If Your Partner Says: We're not using a rubber, and that's it.

You Can Say: OK. You know how to play checkers?

Finally, suppose you are a virgin and have decided to have intercourse and want to use a condom.

If Your Partner Says: Just this once without it. Just the first time.

You'd Better Say: It only takes once to get pregnant. It can only take once to get a sexually transmitted infection.

Don't be afraid of being rejected when you are negotiating for condom use. Remember: When people are given the choice of intercourse with a condom or no intercourse at all, most people will choose to use a condom. Besides, the partner who doesn't care about protecting your health and well-being is not worth your sexual involvement.

Advantages of Using Condoms

Many women and men say they have better sex when they use condoms because they are able to focus on their sexual pleasure without distractions about unintended pregnancy and STIs.

- Condoms allow men to take responsibility for the prevention of unintended pregnancy and sexually transmitted infections.
- Condoms are inexpensive, easy to use, and easily accessible.
- No medical supervision is necessary to use a condom.
- Condoms do not affect a woman's natural hormonal balance.
- Condoms may prevent allergic reactions for a woman who is sensitive to her partner's semen.
- Condoms are lightweight and disposable.
- Condoms are immediately effective and immediately reversible.
- Condoms can help a man stay erect longer.
- Putting on a condom can be part of foreplay.

Disadvantages of Using Condoms

- Men may feel pressured about having to maintain an erection to keep the condoms on.
- Men may feel pressured to ejaculate.
- Condoms may dull sensation for either partner.
- Condoms may interrupt sex play.
- Condoms require high motivation and a strong sense of responsibility.

allergies. They may use animal tissue or plastic condoms instead. Although animal tissue and plastic may not protect as well as latex against viruses like HSV, HPV, HIV, and hepatitis-B, they do offer some protection.

Choosing and Buying a Condom

Condoms usually come rolled, in a ring shape. They may be transparent or opaque, tinted, nipple-ended, rippled, studded, contoured, dry, powdered, or lubricated, with spermicide or without. Usually, size is not marked on the package. But condoms come in different lengths, widths, and thickness. A man may want to try different brands and styles to find out which fits him best. The labels on novelty condoms will provide information about whether or not the condom will protect against pregnancy and STIs.

Nearly as many women as men buy and carry condoms. About 40 percent of all sales of condoms are made to women.

Cost

Condoms are usually available in packages of three or a dozen. Plain, nonlubricated condoms can cost as little as 20 to 30 cents each. Other styles and brands can cost from 60 cents to $2.50 each. For lubricated condoms, the average price per dozen is about $6. Animal tissue and plastic condoms cost about $25 per dozen.

Condoms are available in drugstores, supermarkets, and vending machines. They are also available in Planned Parenthood health centers, other family planning clinics, public health centers, and AIDS service organizations, where they may be less expensive or free.

Female Condom

A female condom, also called a vaginal pouch, is a polyurethane sheath with a flexible ring at each end. It is inserted deep into the vagina like a diaphragm. The ring at the closed end holds the female condom in the vagina. The ring at the open end stays outside the vaginal opening. Female condoms collect semen before, during, and after ejaculation and keep sperm from entering the vagina. They can be used by just about any woman who can use a tampon. Women who are not comfortable touching their genitals probably will not like the female condom.

How Well Female Condoms Work

Of 100 women who use female condoms, 21 will become pregnant during the first year of typical use. Five will become pregnant with perfect use.

The female condom provides protection against many STIs, including HIV. The pouch may offer more protection than a condom against infections such as genital warts and herpes. Since the vulva is partially covered by polyurethane, the female condom protects it more from direct contact with a woman's partner than a male condom does.

How to Use a Female Condom

INSERTING A FEMALE CONDOM

- Lubricate the closed end with any hygienic water- or oil-based lubricant.
- Squeeze together the sides of the inner ring at the closed end and insert the female condom into the vagina like a tampon.
- Push the inner ring with the index finger into the vagina as far as the ring can go—until it reaches the cervix. Be sure to insert the female condom straight into the vagina without twisting it.
- Withdraw your finger and let the outer ring hang about an inch outside the vagina.
- Lubricate the inside of the female condom.

Be sure to guide the penis into the pouch and do not let it slip between the walls of the condom the walls of the vagina. During intercourse, movement of the female condom from side to side is normal. So are some squeaking noises. Using more lubricant can cut down on the noise.

Male and female condoms should not be used at the same time because the friction between them can cause breakage.

Stop intercourse if:

- The penis slips between the walls of the female condom and the walls of the vagina.

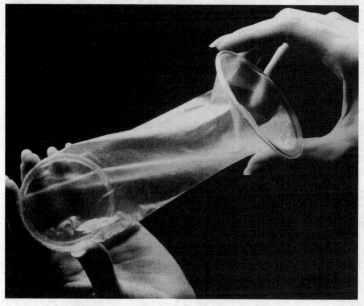

FEMALE CONDOM (VAGINAL POUCH)

- The outer ring is pushed into the vagina.
- The pouch seems to be sticking to or moving with the penis rather than resting in the vagina. In this case, reposition the female condom and put more lubricant inside of it.

Remove the female condom immediately after ejaculation to prevent semen from leaking out.

REMOVING A VAGINAL POUCH

- Squeeze and twist the outer ring to keep the semen inside the female condom.
- Gently pull the female condom out of the vagina.
- Throw the female condom away—but don't flush it down the toilet. Don't use it again, even if intercourse occurs more than once during the same session.

Advantages of Using Female Condoms

- Female condoms are the only method of contraception that allow women to take responsibility for preventing STIs. Women who use them do not have to depend on their partners to wear condoms.
- Men don't have to be erect for the female condom to stay in place.
- Female condoms can be inserted up to eight hours before having sex.
- Female condoms do not affect a woman's natural hormonal balance.
- Made of polyurethane, female condoms can be used by women and men who are allergic to latex.
- Female condoms are immediately effective and immediately reversible.

Disadvantages of Using Female Condoms

- Female condoms are less effective at preventing pregnancy than male condoms.
- Female condoms are more expensive than most male condoms and somewhat harder to find.
- The outer ring of the female condom can slip into the vagina, allowing the penis to thrust between the walls of the condom and the walls of the vagina.
- Some women and men find female condoms messy because they don't hold the semen.
- Female condoms may cause vaginal irritation in some women.
- The outer ring may irritate the vulva.
- The inner ring may irritate the penis.
- Some people say that sensation is reduced.
- Female condoms may squeak during the thrusting of intercourse.

Cost

Female condoms cost about $2.50 each and are sold in packages of three and six. The packaging includes directions for use and packets of lubricant.

Lubricants

When a woman becomes sexually excited, her vagina produces lubrication. It makes intercourse comfortable by making the vagina slippery. Without lubrication, the vagina and penis would become irritated and intercourse would be very unpleasant.

Even more lubrication is needed when partners use male or female condoms. It increases sensation for both partners, keeps the condoms from breaking, and helps keep a female condom in the correct position. There are many brands of lubricants to use with condoms. Many also contain spermicide.

Inserting a drop of lubricant inside the male condom before putting it on is recommended to increase sensation and help the condom slide onto the penis more easily. Applying a drop or two of lubricant to the outside of the condom after putting it on eases entry into the vagina. The lubricant on the outside also reduces the chance that the condom will break during the friction of intercourse. Many condoms are sold already lubricated, but a drop can still be added inside before putting one on.

Lubricating the female condom is also essential even though it is made of tougher materials than the male condom and is less likely to break. Lubricating the outside of the female condom makes it easier to insert. Lubricating the inside increases sensation and keeps it from twisting or getting pulled out or pushed further into the vagina.

Use water-based lubricants with latex condoms, diaphragms, and cervical caps. If water-based lubricants get sticky or dry out, a little water helps make them slippery again. Oil-based lubricants and lubricants that contain alcohol can weaken latex and cause it to break. Use any kind of hygienic lubricant with female condoms or polyurethane or animal tissue male condoms.

Lubricants that can be used with condoms, diaphragms, and cervical caps include H-R® lubricating jelly, Koromex® Gel, K-Y® Lubricating Jelly, Wet®, Ortho-Gynol®, Astroglide®, Surgilube®, contraceptive foams and jellies, and saliva.

Lubricants that can damage latex condoms, diaphragms, and cervical caps include baby oil, hand lotion, cold cream, makeup, massage oil, mineral oil, petroleum jellies—Vaseline®, Bag Balm®—suntan oil, vaginal hormone creams, vaginal medications for yeast infections, hemorrhoid ointments, cooking oils (corn, olive, peanut, and sunflower), and shortenings (butter, margarine, Crisco®, and lard).

◆ Contraceptive Foams, Creams, Jellies, and Suppositories

Contraceptive foams, creams, jellies, and suppositories contain spermicides, chemicals that immobilize sperm and prevent them from joining with an egg. They are inserted deep into the vagina shortly before intercourse. They are used to increase the effectiveness of withdrawal, fertility awareness methods, or other barrier methods by providing backup if a condom breaks or a female condom, diaphragm, or cap becomes dislodged or damaged. Contraceptive creams or jellies must be used when using the diaphragm or cervical cap. Do not rely on these products alone to prevent unintended pregnancy.

Contraceptive foams, creams, jellies, and suppositories are easy to buy in drugstores and some supermarkets. No prescriptions or fittings are needed. Once learned, insertion is easy and may be done by a partner as part of sex play.

Contraceptive foams, creams, jellies, and suppositories combined with other behavioral or barrier methods are especially suitable for women who:

- do not have intercourse often
- are breast-feeding
- will not or cannot go to a clinic or physician
- need a backup method if they forget to take the Pill
- want to increase the effectiveness of the condom
- need a backup method until their diaphragms or caps are refitted
- need a backup method until their IUDs are repositioned

How Well These Methods Work for Contraception

Of 100 women who use contraceptive foams, creams, jellies, or suppositories, 26 will become pregnant during the first year of typical use. Six will become pregnant with perfect use. Using a condom increases effectiveness.

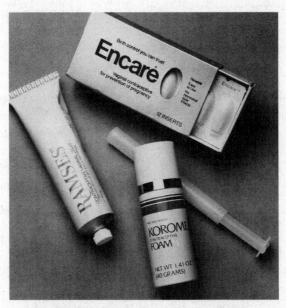

CONTRACEPTIVE FOAMS, CREAMS, JELLIES, AND SUPPOSITORIES

The effectiveness rates of all barrier methods improve with continued use. As with any contraceptive, the manufacturer's directions, supplied in each package insert, should be read, understood, and followed.

Spermicide and Sexually Transmitted Infections

The spermicides in contraceptive foams, creams, jellies, and suppositories offer some protection against gonorrhea, chlamydia, and trichomoniasis. By reducing risk of these STIs, these methods provide some protection against pelvic inflammatory disease (PID), a serious infection of the reproductive tract. Preventing PID reduces the possibility of infertility and ectopic pregnancy.

Some health care professionals believe that the spermicide nonoxynol-9, contained in contraceptive foams and other products, offers some protection against HIV. Many others maintain that spermicide may actually increase the risk of infection by irritating the vaginal lining.

How to Use Contraceptive Foam

Contraceptive foam comes in an aerosol can. Each package contains an applicator. The pressurized gases in the can make the foam bubble when it is put into the applicator. The bubbles help the spermicide cover the cervix and spread evenly throughout the vagina. Some foams come in prefilled, easy-to-carry applicators. (A woman who is uncomfortable about touching her vagina in order to

> In the mid-1980s, there was some concern about the effect of products containing spermicides on fetal development. However, scientific study of more than 4,500 infants showed no connection between the use of vaginal barrier methods and birth defects.

insert a contraceptive may prefer this method because of the easy-to-use applicator.)

INSERTING THE FOAM

- Shake the container at least 20 times before using. Shaking creates more bubbles in the foam. More bubbles form a better and stronger barrier throughout the crevices of the vagina. Check the manufacturer's instructions to see if more than one application is necessary and when each application should be made—when in doubt, use more.

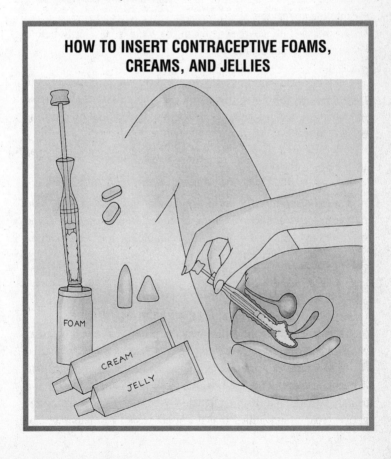

HOW TO INSERT CONTRACEPTIVE FOAMS, CREAMS, AND JELLIES

- Fill the applicator according to the instructions included in the packaging. The foam applicator consists of a cylinder and a plunger. It works the way a tampon applicator does.
- Lie down, squat, or put one foot up on a chair, and insert the applicator as deeply into the vagina as is comfortable.
- Withdraw the applicator one-half inch so that foam is deposited in front of the cervix.
- Slowly push the plunger to release the foam evenly.
- Remove the applicator from the vagina, keeping the plunger pressed into the applicator to prevent drawing the foam back into the applicator.
- To increase effectiveness, put in the foam very shortly before each act of intercourse.

The bubbles begin to go flat in about 30 minutes. As the foam dries out, it becomes less effective. Insert more foam if intercourse continues beyond 30 minutes. A fresh application of foam is required for each act of vaginal intercourse.

Lie back for a short while after intercourse for assurance that as much foam as possible lies against the cervix.

Do not douche for at least eight hours after intercourse.

Unless disposable, clean the applicator and plunger with soap and warm water and store it with the foam. Both should be stored away from extreme heat or cold. For example, do not keep foam on a radiator or in a refrigerator.

How to Use
Contraceptive Creams and Jellies

Contraceptive creams and jellies may not produce as much liquid as foams and may be less messy. Although most are designed to be used with a diaphragm or cervical cap, some manufacturers package them with applicators to be used without either. Planned Parenthood strongly urges that a male or female condom be used with contraceptive creams and jellies that are used without a diaphragm or cervical cap.

Follow the directions on the package insert for filling the applicator unless the applicator is prefilled and disposable.

INSERTING CONTRACEPTIVE CREAM OR JELLY

- Lie down, squat, or put one foot up on a chair, and insert the applicator as deeply into the vagina as is comfortable. It works the way a tampon applicator does.
- Withdraw the applicator approximately one-half inch so that the cream or jelly is most likely to be deposited in front of the cervix, not squeezed to the sides.
- Slowly push the plunger all the way into the applicator to release the contents evenly.
- Remove the applicator from the vagina, keeping the plunger pressed into the applicator to prevent drawing the cream or jelly back into the applicator.
- A fresh application of cream or jelly is required for each act of vaginal intercourse. Reapply if vaginal intercourse continues beyond 30 minutes.
- Wash the applicator and plunger in warm water and store for future use. Disposable applicators should be thrown away out of the reach of children.

Women who like to douche should wait at least eight hours after the last act of vaginal intercourse.

How to Use
Contraceptive Suppositories

Contraceptive suppositories are capsules, tablets, or films containing spermicide that melt into a liquid after being placed deep in the vagina. Effervescing suppositories are also available. The bubbles created within the vagina by effervescing suppositories help to provide a physical as well as chemical barrier to the sperm.

For some women, suppositories are easier to insert than the applicators for other vaginal contraceptives. Suppositories also tend to be less messy than foam.

Some women experience a sensation of warmth when effervescing suppositories dissolve. Some like it, others don't. Suppositories do not require removal because they melt into liquids that are washed away with normal vaginal secretions.

INSERTING A CONTRACEPTIVE SUPPOSITORY

- Follow the instructions on the package insert.
- Handle and insert the suppository with clean hands.
- Use an index finger to slip the suppository deep into the vagina, as close to the cervix as possible. Some suppositories are packaged in disposable applicators.
- Insert quickly because if the suppository begins to melt, it may stick to the fingers and become difficult to position correctly.
- Make sure that the suppository has completely dissolved by waiting the amount of time indicated on the package insert (usually 10 to 15 minutes) before beginning intercourse or before the penis touches the vagina.
- Use at least one suppository for each act of intercourse.

Caution: Do not crumple suppository film into a ball for insertion. It may take longer to dissolve in that shape and may not position correctly. For insertion, drape the film over the index finger as directed in the packaging instructions.

The effectiveness of the suppository decreases rapidly after 30 minutes. If vaginal intercourse has not been completed 45 minutes after inserting the suppository, insert another into the vagina and wait 15 minutes before resuming intercourse.

A woman using a contraceptive suppository should not douche for at least eight hours after intercourse.

Caution: Be sure the suppository package is marked "contraceptive" or "birth control." Do not take contraceptive suppositories orally. Do not insert into the urethra.

Planned Parenthood strongly urges that male or female condoms be used with contraceptive suppositories.

Advantages of Contraceptive Foams, Creams, Jellies, and Suppositories

- They are sold over the counter and do not require medical examination, supervision, or follow-up.
- They are inexpensive and easy to use.
- They offer some protection against chlamydia, gonorrhea, trichomoniasis, and PID.
- They can be inserted as part of sex play.
- Products can be combined. If a woman has only a little left of one brand, she can use it with some of another.
- They do not affect a woman's natural hormonal balance.
- They do not cause known medical side effects, unless a woman or her partner has an unusual allergy.
- They can provide extra lubrication for women.
- They are immediately effective and immediately reversible.
- They are not toxic—except to sperm.

Disadvantages of Contraceptive Foams, Creams, Jellies, and Suppositories

- Spermicides have relatively high failure rates when used alone and should be used with other methods of birth control.
- Some women and men find them messy.
- Some women and men develop skin irritations.
- Reapplication can interrupt sex play.
- People who enjoy oral sex may object to the taste of contraceptive foam. They may choose to insert the foam after oral sex but before the penis touches the vulva or vaginal intercourse begins. Although some spermicides are flavored, partners may dislike the way that spermicide numbs their tongues.

Side Effects of Contraceptive Foams, Creams, Jellies, and Suppositories

Between 2 and 4 percent of men and women are sensitive to the spermicides in contraceptive foams, creams, jellies, and suppositories. They may develop genital irritation and itching. They may be less sensitive to a different product or brand.

The spermicide in contraceptive foams, creams, jellies, and suppositories may alter the bacterial environment of the vagina. This may increase a woman's risk of developing bacterial vaginosis (vaginitis) or vaginal candidiasis (yeast infections).

Cost

Contraceptive foams, creams, jellies, and suppositories can be purchased in drugstores, supermarkets, and women's health and family planning centers.

Disposable, prefilled applicators of foams, creams, and jellies cost about $1 per application. Kits that are packaged with reusable applicators may be less expensive per application. Kits of foam or jelly that contain an applicator cost from $8 to $18. The applicator can be saved and refill tubes of jelly bought for $4 to $8. The cost of foam refills and containers is usually under $10. Large cans of foam contain about 20 to 40 applications.

Suppositories are sold in packages of 12, 20, or 36. The cost may be as low as $4 a package. Packets of 12 squares of film are available for about $7. Costs may be reduced in public health centers and family planning clinics.

> **Caution:** Drugstores and supermarkets often shelve vaginal contraceptive foam and feminine deodorants side by side. Products purchased for birth control should be clearly marked "contraceptive" or "birth control." So-called feminine hygiene products offer no protection against pregnancy or STIs. Consult the pharmacist if the labeling is not clear.

Diaphragm and Cervical Cap

Diaphragms and cervical caps are soft latex barriers that cover the cervix. Both must be used with a contraceptive cream or jelly. The diaphragm is a shallow, dome-shaped cup with a flexible rim. It fits in the vagina and over the cervix. The cervical cap is thimble-shaped and smaller than the diaphragm. It fits snugly onto the cervix.

Diaphragms and caps keep sperm from joining with the egg. They block the opening to the uterus and prevent sperm from entering. The contraceptive cream or jelly applied to the diaphragm or cap immobilizes sperm.

Choosing a Diaphragm or Cervical Cap

Diaphragms and caps are available by prescription only. A pelvic examination by a clinician is needed to determine the correct size. The clinician will also provide instruction for use, insertion, and removal.

Diaphragms are available in a wide variety of sizes. Three different types of flexible rims are also available: arcing spring, flat spring, and coil spring.

The arcing spring rim is popular with many women because it tends to be easy to insert. One type of diaphragm with an arcing spring rim can be folded at any point along the rim. Two other types can be folded at only two points and are less likely to unfold during insertion.

The second type of rim, the coil spring rim, has a spiral of wire inside and provides somewhat more pressure to hold the diaphragm in place. The coil spring is useful for women with relaxed vaginal muscle tone—especially after the vaginal delivery of a baby, a time when vaginal muscle tone is very relaxed.

Arcing spring and coil spring rims are also available in wide seal versions. They have an extra flange of soft latex inside the outer rim. The flange improves the seal and holds the spermicide more completely against the cervix.

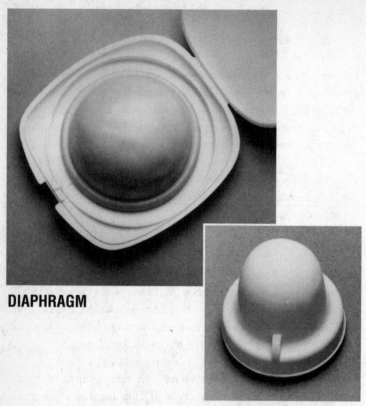

DIAPHRAGM

CERVICAL CAP

The oldest type of rim is the flat spring rim, which has a metal band inside. The flat spring places minimal pressure on the vagina and is often most appropriate for women who have never given birth.

The prescription of which type to use depends on the size of the vagina and the strength of the vaginal muscles. A woman may want to ask her health care provider why her particular diaphragm was chosen for her, so that she will understand what to expect and will know what to look for if she needs to choose another type.

Cervical caps are available in only four sizes and may need to be refitted in certain circumstances. The rims of caps are hard rubber and do not contain metal springs.

Who Can Use Diaphragms or Cervical Caps

Diaphragms can be used by most women. They are not appropriate for women who have:

- poor vaginal muscle tone
- a tipped uterus or a sagging (prolapsed) uterus
- vaginal obstructions, such as a cystocele (bulging of the walls of the bladder), a rectocele (bulging of the walls of the rectum), or vaginal stenosis (narrowing of the vaginal canal)
- a history of toxic shock syndrome (a rare but potentially dangerous disease caused by infection and most common in menstruating women)
- recurrent urinary tract infections
- allergies or sensitivities to latex or spermicides

Cervical caps can be used by most women. They are not appropriate if the correct size is unavailable, if a woman finds insertion too difficult, or if a woman has:

- an abnormal Pap test
- a history of toxic shock syndrome
- a sexually transmitted or reproductive tract infection
- inflammation of the cervix

A woman should not use the diaphragm or cap if she is using a medication or preparation that contains an oil-based product such as Vaseline. It can cause latex to deteriorate. And the diaphragm and cap should not be used during menstruation.

Women with very short menstrual cycles also should not rely on the diaphragm or cap. If ovulation occurs within five or six days of the last day of menstruation, sperm from intercourse during menstruation may fertilize the egg.

How Well Diaphragms and Cervical Caps Work

Of 100 women using diaphragms, about 20 will become pregnant during the first year of typical use. Six will become pregnant with perfect use.

The Pap Test and the Cervical Cap

A woman must have normal results from a Pap test and pelvic exam before she can use a cervical cap. The clinician takes a smear for the Pap test on the day of the fitting unless the results of a recent test are available. If the test results are abnormal, the woman will be unable to use the cap until further testing shows normal results. Her clinician will let her know if additional testing or treatment is necessary.

A follow-up visit is necessary approximately three months after the fitting. At that time, the fit is checked and another Pap test is done to check for any changes in the cervical cells. The U.S. Food and Drug Administration (FDA) requires two Pap tests within a short time. This is because studies performed by the National Institutes of Health for the FDA showed abnormal Pap results after three months among 4 percent of women who used the cervical cap. Fewer of the women (1.7 percent) who used diaphragms in those studies had abnormal results. After six months of use, the rates of abnormal test results were about the same for women using diaphragms and those using caps.

Because women using the diaphragm or cervical cap may be more likely to develop cell changes, it is safer for those whose Pap tests are not entirely normal to use another method of contraception.

Women who have given birth may have unacceptably high failure rates using the cervical cap. Of 100 women using cervical caps who have never given birth, about 20 will become pregnant during the first year of typical use. Nine will become pregnant with perfect use.

Of 100 women using cervical caps who have given birth, about 40 will become pregnant during the first year of typical use. About 26 will become pregnant with perfect use.

To increase effectiveness, a couple should do the following:

- Check to be sure that the diaphragm or cap covers the cervix before vaginal intercourse every time.
- Use a fresh application of contraceptive cream or jelly if intercourse is repeated.
- Use a condom during the woman's most fertile times.
- Use a backup method of birth control for at least the first full month of use and the first few acts of intercourse with a new partner. Different sexual positions, penis sizes, and thrusting techniques and angles may dislodge the diaphragm or cap.
- Move the diaphragm or cap back into place if it slips out of place during intercourse, unless the man has ejaculated. If the man has ejaculated, remove the diaphragm or cap, wash it, and reinsert it with a new application of spermicide. If this happens during a time when the woman may be fertile, she may want to contact her clinician immediately to discuss emergency contraception.
- Never douche when the diaphragm or cervical cap is in place. The douche may wash away the spermicide or push it into the cervix.

Women should have pelvic examinations once a year. During these annual examinations, the diaphragm or cervical cap can be checked for wear and size. A different size diaphragm may be needed after a full-term pregnancy, abdominal or pelvic surgery, or miscarriage or abortion after 14 weeks of pregnancy.

The spermicides in contraceptive creams and jellies used with diaphragms and caps offer some protection against gonorrhea, chlamydia, and trichomoniasis. By reducing risk for these STIs, diaphragms and cervical caps provide some protection against pelvic inflammatory disease. Preventing PID reduces the chance of infertility and ectopic pregnancy.

Some health care professionals believe the spermicide also offers protection against HIV. Others maintain that spermicide may actually increase the risk of infection by irritating the vaginal lining.

Because diaphragms and cervical caps cover the cervix, an area that's highly vulnerable to irritation and infection during intercourse, they may help a woman reduce the risk of genital tract infections and cervical cancer.

How to Use a Diaphragm

A diaphragm may be inserted up to six hours before intercourse.

INSERTING A DIAPHRAGM

- Wash hands with soap and warm water.
- Put about a teaspoonful of contraceptive cream or jelly in the cup of the diaphragm and spread some around the rim. Use a dot of the cream or jelly to lubricate the outside rim to help glide the diaphragm into place. Vaseline or cold cream should never be used because they damage rubber and do not affect sperm.
- Find a comfortable position—stand with one foot on a chair, sit on the edge of a chair, lie down, or squat.
- Separate the labia with one hand and with the other pinch the rim of the diaphragm to fold it in half. Then place the index finger in the center of the fold for a firmer grip. The contraceptive cream or jelly must be inside the fold.

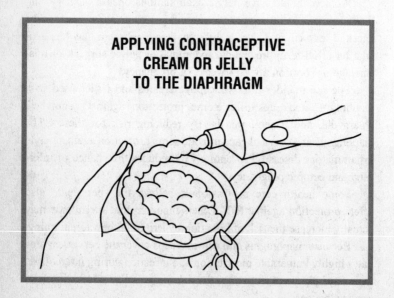

**APPLYING CONTRACEPTIVE
CREAM OR JELLY
TO THE DIAPHRAGM**

USING A DIAPHRAGM

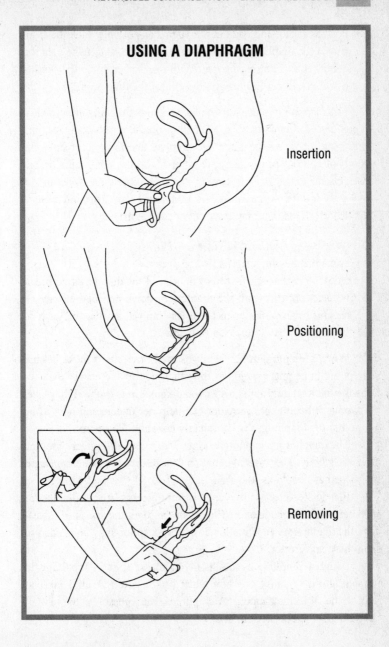

Insertion

Positioning

Removing

- Push as far up and back in the vagina as possible, tuck the front rim of the diaphragm behind the pubic bone, and make sure the cervix is covered by the rim. With one finger, trace the outline of the entire cervix through the cup of the diaphragm.

The diaphragm must stay in place six to eight hours after the last intercourse. If intercourse is repeated or occurs more than six hours after insertion, leave the diaphragm in place and insert another application of contraceptive cream, jelly, or foam into the vagina before intercourse begins. Do not leave in place for more than 24 hours.

A thin sanitary napkin worn for an hour or two after intercourse can absorb fluids that may flow out of the vagina.

REMOVING A DIAPHRAGM

- Wash hands with soap and warm water.
- Hook a finger over the top of the rim of the diaphragm to break the suction; then pull the diaphragm down and out. It may be helpful to sit on an open toilet for removal so that the gush of spermicide that is released falls into it.

When a diaphragm has been inserted properly, it tucks behind the pubic bone and extends to the other side of the cervix. Always check with a finger to make sure the diaphragm is in the right place. A woman's health care provider can help her understand how to be sure that the diaphragm is completely covering the cervix.

The diaphragm cannot become loose and disappear into the woman's body. The vaginal canal ends at the cervix. The diaphragm is placed as deeply as it can go.

Plastic inserters, also called introducers, are available for women who may have short fingers or can't get the knack of inserting the diaphragm. In some locales, a prescription may be needed to purchase an inserter.

Using a diaphragm should be painless. If it is too large, a diaphragm may cause pressure when it is inserted. A clinician can check the fit if this happens. A diaphragm that presses on the rectum should also be checked for size.

How to Use a Cervical Cap

The cervical cap can be inserted up to 40 hours before intercourse.

INSERTING A CERVICAL CAP

- Wash hands with soap and warm water.
- Fill the dome of the cervical cap one-third full of spermicide. Avoid getting any on the rim—it could interfere with the suction needed to keep the cap in place.
- Find a comfortable position—stand with one foot on a chair, sit on the edge of a chair, lie down, or squat.
- Locate the cervix with the index and middle fingers.
- Separate the labia with one hand and squeeze the cap rim together with the other.
- Hold the cap dome-side down, slide it into the vagina, and push it up and onto the cervix. Use the forefinger and middle finger to complete the insertion, pushing the cap toward the back wall of the vagina until it covers the cervix.
- Press the rim into place on the cervix, pinch the rounded end to create suction, then twist the cap like a jar lid.
- Sweep a finger around the cap to make sure the cervix is completely covered and there are no gaps. A small part of the cervix outside the cap will feel like a small bump. Try to eliminate the bump by pushing the cap more firmly onto the cervix. If that doesn't work, remove the cap and start again. If the spermicide has oozed out, it will be necessary to add more. If spermicide has gotten onto the rim, wipe it dry.

Wait 10 to 20 minutes before having intercourse to let the rim of the cap develop adequate suction. The cap can cause low back pain or menstrual-type cramping if it is too tight. A clinician can check the fit if this happens.

The cap must stay in place eight hours after the last intercourse. It should not remain in place for a total of more than 48 hours. Do not douche with the cap in place.

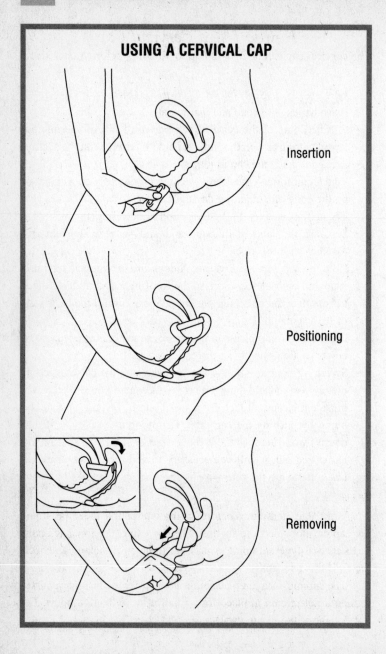

USING A CERVICAL CAP

Insertion

Positioning

Removing

REMOVING A CERVICAL CAP

- Wash hands with soap and warm water.
- Push the rim away from the cervix with one or two fingers to break the suction.
- Hook one finger under the rim and pull the cap out.

A woman who has trouble putting the cap in place may try insertion while squatting and bearing down as if she were having a bowel movement. This position pushes the cervix down farther into the vaginal canal, enabling her to reach it more easily. This position may also be helpful for removing the cap. Plastic diaphragm inserters can help remove a cervical cap.

Check the position of the cap before each act of intercourse. Move it back into place if it has become dislodged. Slippage may mean a poor fit, especially if the cap has been used properly for a while. A clinician can check the fit of a cap that slips.

Women who use cervical caps should use a different form of birth control for eight weeks after having a cervical biopsy or pelvic surgery or until any reproductive tract infection has cleared up and their clinicians have advised resuming cap use.

Care of Diaphragms and Cervical Caps

Diaphragms and caps can last about two years with proper care. Latex deteriorates with time and use. Washing it with harsh detergents, disinfectants, or other strong cleaners can reduce its life. The FDA suggests that diaphragms and caps be replaced every year.

- After removal, wash the diaphragm or cap with mild antibacterial or nonallergenic soap and warm water—no detergents or perfumed soap.
- Let the diaphragm or cap dry on a clean surface in the open air. Place it to dry on its open case away from strong light or heat.
- Do not use powders—they can cause infections. Scented powders and oil-based lubricants, such as Vaseline, can damage latex.
- Examine the diaphragm or cervical cap regularly for small holes or weak spots. Pin holes can be spotted by holding the

Practice Makes Perfect

The better a diaphragm or cervical cap fits and is inserted, the better it will stay in place and the better it will protect against pregnancy. A woman's clinician should watch her insert and remove the diaphragm or cap after she is fitted to be sure she is doing it correctly. She should practice inserting and removing it at home, too, in order to be confident and relaxed when she uses it with a partner.

diaphragm up to the light and stretching the rubber gently between the fingers. If a hole is discovered, no matter how tiny, another method of birth control must be used until the diaphragm or cap can be replaced.

Keep the diaphragm or cervical cap clean at all times. If it develops an offensive odor, wash it thoroughly with mild soap and warm water. The groove inside the cap requires special attention. Turning the cap inside out may make it easier to clean. Use a cotton-tipped swab to clean the groove.

Diaphragms and caps can still be used if the rubber becomes discolored. If the rubber puckers, however, especially near the rim, it has become dangerously thin. If the material feels sticky or slimy even after being cleaned, it's probably time for a new one.

Check the diaphragm or cervical cap for holes or deterioration and clean it if it has not been used for a while.

Side Effects

Some women who use diaphragms develop frequent bladder infections. The symptoms include frequent urination and burning sensations. Infection is not always the cause. Sometimes the diaphragm presses against and irritates the urethra. A woman should report such symptoms to her clinician. A woman who suffers recurrent bladder infections may be advised to:

- urinate before inserting the diaphragm
- urinate after intercourse
- be refitted
- try a diaphragm with a different rim

Recurrent urinary tract infections can be painful and lead to more serious infections. If none of these suggestions offers relief, a clinician will suggest the woman choose another method of birth control.

The spermicides used with diaphragms and cervical caps may alter the bacterial environment of the vagina. This may increase a woman's risk of developing bacterial vaginosis (vaginitis) or vaginal candidiasis (yeast infections).

Rarely, abnormal cell growth occurs in the cervix during the first

---

Toxic Shock Syndrome

Rare cases of toxic shock syndrome (TSS) have been reported with diaphragm use. The symptoms of TSS include:
- sudden high fever
- diarrhea
- vomiting
- sore throat, aching muscles and joints
- dizziness, faintness, weakness
- a sunburnlike rash

If such symptoms occur, a woman should remove the diaphragm or cervical cap and contact her health care provider immediately.

Some women use diaphragms or cervical caps to collect menstrual flow during their periods. Planned Parenthood does not recommend the use of the diaphragm or cap for this purpose because it increases the risk of TSS. Likewise, diaphragms and caps should not be used during menstruation or any other vaginal bleeding.

Contact your clinician if:

- You have trouble inserting or removing your diaphragm or cervical cap.
- You spot signs of wear other than slight discoloration on your diaphragm or cap, such as a hole, tear, or crack of any size, or stickiness after cleaning.
- You experience pain during intercourse—or your partner does.
- You experience pain or discomfort when the diaphragm or cap is in place.
- You develop an unpleasant vaginal odor or an unusual vaginal discharge.
- You think that you may be pregnant.
- You experience the symptoms associated with toxic shock syndrome. Remove your diaphragm or cervical cap and call your health care provider immediately.
- You find that your diaphragm or cap seems to be fitting differently than before.
- You discover that your diaphragm or cap slips during intercourse or when you exercise, cough, or strain. Such slippage may be caused by deterioration of the cap or intercourse with a new partner.
- You feel genital burning or irritation while the cap is in place—or your partner does.
- You discover blood on or inside your diaphragm or cap when you take it out, and you are not menstruating.
- You develop a burning sensation while urinating.
- You develop irritation or itching in the genital area.
- You have irregular spotting or bleeding.

few months of cap use. The condition, which would normally be detected with a Pap test, usually corrects itself but sometimes requires medical treatment.

Some people experience genital irritation from diaphragms and cervical caps. Some women experience mild vaginal irritation and some men experience mild penile irritation from the spermicide used *with* diaphragms and cervical caps. Spermicides are made with different formulas. If one brand is irritating, a couple may try another. If the rim is causing irritation, they may try a different style.

A woman who is allergic to latex should not try to use a diaphragm or cervical cap. Allergic reactions to latex can be very serious.

Contraceptive jellies may be less likely to contribute to the development of unpleasant vaginal odors than contraceptive creams. If an odor problem persists, it may be that the diaphragm or cap has been left inside the body for too long. It should be washed with warm water and soap. If the unpleasant vaginal odor or unusual discharge continues, a vaginal infection may have developed. If so, the woman should contact her clinician.

Where to Get Diaphragms and Cervical Caps and What They Cost

Diaphragms and cervical caps are available from Planned Parenthood, other women's health centers, university and college health services, and private medical practices. Women's health centers and nurse practitioners may be more likely than physicians to offer cervical caps.

Diaphragms and caps may be purchased with a prescription at a drugstore or clinic. An examination costs $50 to $200. Diaphragms and caps average $15 to $50. A tube of contraceptive cream or jelly usually costs $8 to $17. It contains enough spermicide for about 10 uses of a diaphragm or about 30 uses of a cervical cap. Medicaid covers these costs. Private health insurance coverage for birth control varies.

The nearest Planned Parenthood health center can be contacted for more information about cervical caps or diaphragms. Call 800-230-PLAN. Another source of information is Cervical Cap Ltd., the sole U.S. distributor of cervical caps to health care providers. To contact: Cervical Cap Ltd., 430 Monterey Ave., Suite 1B, Los Gatos, CA 95030; 408-395-2100.

Advantages of Using Diaphragms or Cervical Caps

- Diaphragms and cervical caps offer some protection against certain STIs, including gonorrhea and chlamydia.
- They offer some protection against pelvic inflammatory disease (PID).
- Diaphragms may reduce a woman's risk of developing cervical cancer.
- They do not interfere with a woman's natural hormonal balance.
- They generally cannot be felt by either partner.
- They can be carried conveniently in pocket or purse.
- They can be used during breast-feeding.
- They are immediately effective and immediately reversible.
- They do not interrupt sex play if inserted ahead of time.
- Spermicide used with diaphragms increases lubrication. (The spermicide in the cap remains in the cap and does not provide lubrication.)

Disadvantages of Using Diaphragms or Cervical Caps

- It may be difficult for some women to insert diaphragms or cervical caps.
- A woman must be willing to insert the diaphragm or cap every time she has vaginal intercourse.
- Diaphragms require refitting every year or two to see if a different size is needed.
- Diaphragms may become dislodged if the woman is on top during intercourse.
- Cervical caps, when used by women who have given birth, have a very high failure rate.
- The possibility of developing side effects associated with diaphragms or cervical caps may be unacceptable.

Latex Allergy

The sap of the rubber tree and its synthetic version are both called latex. Products made of latex are often called "natural rubber products." Most condoms and diaphragms and cervical caps are natural rubber products. People who are allergic to latex should not use any of these methods. Their allergic reactions to latex can range from mild to life-threatening.

From 2 to 7 percent of people are allergic to latex, which has only recently been recognized as an allergen. The growing prevalence and awareness of latex allergies is attributed to the increased use of latex gloves. Nurses, surgeons, laboratory workers, food service workers, and others who use thin surgical-type gloves on the job are at particular risk. Anyone who has ever had even a mild reaction to eating bananas, avocados, or chestnuts may be allergic to latex as well—these fruits and nuts are related to rubber trees.

In its 1992 recommendations to health professionals, the American College of Allergy, Asthma, and Immunology listed several possible indications of latex allergy—especially if any of the symptoms are associated with wearing latex gloves in the workplace:

- worsening red skin rash (eczema)
- hives
- eye infections (conjunctivitis)
- runny nose
- symptoms of asthma—wheezing and difficulty in breathing

A common reaction to latex is contact dermatitis, an itchy, scaly, uncomfortable rash resembling those caused by poison ivy. The rash appears where the body had contact with latex. Latex may be the culprit if a man's penis or a woman's vagina itches 12 to 24 hours after having contact with a condom, diaphragm, or cervical cap.

The most serious, though rare, allergic reaction to latex is an anaphylactic reaction (anaphylaxis). During such a reaction, the victim's throat can quickly swell and constrict the windpipe, making it

Are You Allergic to Latex?

As with many allergies, the symptoms of latex allergy can grow worse with every exposure. This phenomenon is called increased sensitivity. Having a mild reaction at first does not mean that everything will be OK. In fact, if you have any reaction at all, it's likely that the reaction will be more severe the next time.

Contact a knowledgeable health professional—an allergist is the best bet—if you notice swelling, redness, and itching in the area of your body that has had contact with a latex product. For example, your lips or mouth may be affected after blowing up a balloon or after having your teeth examined or cleaned by a dentist or dental hygienist wearing latex gloves. Your vagina or rectum may be affected after being examined by your health care provider or after you have used latex condoms for sexual intercourse. Or you may develop red, itchy hands, a runny nose, nasal congestion, or signs of asthma after using latex gloves for household chores.

impossible for that person to breathe. Early warning signals for ana-phylaxis include a tingling feeling, flushed skin, a rash, and dizzi-ness. Medical help should be called immediately.

Clinicians may have difficulty spotting the milder symptoms of latex allergy. Not all laboratories are equipped to test for it. Skin tests are less definitive than for other allergies, and blood tests for this allergy are also imprecise. Anyone with symptoms should describe them in detail to an allergist—preferably one who has had experience with latex allergies.

The medication used to treat allergic reactions to latex is injectable epinephrine (adrenaline—Ana-Kit® or EpiPen®). It is also used by people who are allergic to insect bites and certain foods. Syringes prefilled with medication should be kept on hand at all times for emergency use by those with severe allergies. Antihistamine nose sprays may offer some relief in a pinch while someone calls for emergency help. Anyone with a potentially life threatening allergy should be sure to wear a special I.D. bracelet.

The best "treatment" for latex allergy is prevention—staying away from latex. Anyone who thinks he or she has a latex allergy should stay clear of latex contraceptives and sex toys until allergies can be ruled out.

People who are allergic to latex and want protection against STIs can use plastic or animal tissue condoms or vaginal pouches. While these barriers may not offer as effective protection as latex, the protection that is offered is still significant.

6

◆

Reversible Contraception— Intrauterine Devices (IUDs)

- *What IUDs Are*

Intrauterine devices, commonly called IUDs, are the world's most popular method of reversible birth control for women. When placed inside a woman's uterus, an IUD helps prevent pregnancy. Nearly 100 million women use IUDs, 20 percent of all women who use birth control, including 40 percent of the women in China who use contraception. Intrauterine devices are the least expensive reversible method of contraception available by prescription.

Intrauterine devices are recognized by the World Health Organization and the American Medical Association as one of the safest and most effective temporary methods of birth control for women. Unfortunately, several years of negative publicity and speculation following lawsuits brought on by the sale and use of a faulty IUD—the Dalkon Shield®—raised many questions about the safety of all IUDs. Lawsuits sparked by the Dalkon Shield caused some manufacturers to withdraw even safe IUDs from the American market. For these reasons, the variety of available IUDs in the United States is limited, and the once popular method is used by fewer than 2 percent of American women who use reversible contraception.

◆

What IUDs Are

An IUD is a small device made of firm but flexible plastic that is fit inside the uterus to provide reversible birth control. A string attached to the IUD hangs through the opening of the cervix when the IUD is in place. The string is used to check the position of the IUD and to remove it when necessary.

Intrauterine devices are available by prescription only. A health care professional helps the woman decide which is the right type for her and inserts it in her uterus. Once inserted, the IUD is immediately effective. When removed, its contraceptive effect is immediately reversed.

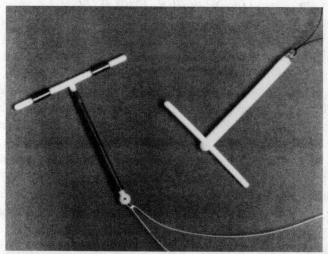

PARAGARD® (COPPER T 380A) AND PROGESTASERT®

Not all IUDs are alike. There are several types, and they come in different sizes. Two types are currently available in the United States. One type, the ParaGard® Copper T 380A, contains copper and can be left in place for 10 years. The other, the Progestasert®, continuously releases a small amount of progestin and must be replaced every year.

How IUDs Work

Intrauterine devices primarily work by preventing fertilization of the egg, though scientists are not entirely sure why. The devices seem to affect the way the sperm or egg moves. It may be that substances released by IUDs immobilize sperm or that IUDs prompt the egg to move through the fallopian tube too fast to be fertilized.

The progestin in the Progestasert also thickens cervical mucus, providing a barrier that prevents sperm from entering the uterus. Furthermore, it affects the lining of the uterus in ways that would prevent implantation in the unlikely event that an egg is fertilized.

The Structure of an IUD

Both IUDs available in the United States are made of polyethylene in a T-shape about an inch-and-a-half tall. In both brands, the polyethylene is coated with barium, a metal used to make the IUD clearly visible with an X ray.

The year's supply of progestin in the Progestasert IUD is stored in a reservoir in the stem of the T. The hormone affects only the reproductive tract. Only a very minute amount of the hormone enters the woman's bloodstream.

A fine copper wire is wound around the stem of the ParaGard Copper T 380A, and more copper is embedded in its crossbar. The copper adds to the effectiveness of this IUD in two ways. It affects the behavior of enzymes in the lining of the uterus to prevent implantation. It also causes the production of increased amounts of prostaglandins—fatty acids that affect the hormones that support pregnancy.

Both IUDs have a strong plastic monofilament—a string—that is threaded through a hole in the bottom of the T and tied in half with a knot. The string cannot absorb, or "wick," fluid or bacteria into the uterus the way a cotton string would.

The string has two purposes. It allows for easier removal by a health care professional when the time comes. The string also allows a woman to know if her IUD is still in the correct position. If the string seems to shorten or lengthen, the IUD may have moved out of place. If the string can't be located, it may mean that contractions of the uterus during menstruation or sex play have expelled the IUD.

Who Can Use IUDs

An IUD may be right for a woman if:

- She has had a baby and her family is complete.
- She has only one sex partner who has sex only with her. Intrauterine devices do not protect against sexually transmitted infections (STIs). A woman who uses an IUD must use condoms if she has more than one sex partner—or has a partner who has more than one partner. Otherwise, she is at high risk of developing pelvic inflammatory disease (PID), which can scar the reproductive organs and cause infertility.
- She wants a very effective, long-term, reversible method of birth control.
- She is breast-feeding.
- She has no history of PID.
- She has access to medical care if problems develop.
- She cannot use hormonal methods such as the Pill because she smokes or has certain conditions such as high blood pressure.
- Her uterus is large enough to accommodate an IUD.

A woman should not use an IUD if she might be pregnant or if:

- She has a sexually transmitted infection such as chlamydia or gonorrhea.
- She has a history of pelvic infection that has impaired her fertility.

- She has had an inflammation of the lining of the uterus after giving birth or an infected abortion in the past three months.
- She has untreated or uncontrolled acute cervicitis or vaginitis, including bacterial vaginosis.
- She has abnormal vaginal bleeding.
- She has conditions associated with increased susceptibility to infections with microorganisms, including leukemia, AIDS, and intravenous drug use.
- She has certain anatomical abnormalities of the cervix, uterus, or ovaries that would make insertion difficult or dangerous.
- She has abnormal Pap test results or cancer of the uterus or cervix.
- She has actinomycosis, a bacterial infection of the reproductive tract.
- She has a previously inserted IUD that has not been removed.
- She has a uterus that is shorter or smaller than the IUD.
- She has no access to medical care if problems develop.

Copper IUDs should not be used by women who are allergic to copper; have Wilson's disease, a rare hereditary disorder associated with the accumulation of potentially dangerous amounts of copper in body tissues; or are undergoing physical therapy techniques involving use of heat (diathermy) to transmit energy into deep tissues. The concern with diathermy is that the copper in an IUD could become hot enough to burn tissue in the uterus and lead to scarring.

Special evaluations must be made for women who have a history of heart disease or certain other conditions. These conditions include valvular heart disease, the use of an artificial heart valve, or ventricular or atrial septal defects (defects in the wall dividing the chambers of the heart) that have not been repaired. There is a possibility that an infection associated with an IUD in a woman with one of these conditions could lead to bacterial endocarditis, a very dangerous infection of the heart and blood.

Because some women have physical or medical conditions that may rule out IUD use, a pelvic examination and a complete medical history are important. The physical examination will let the practitioner know if a woman's cervix, vagina, and internal organs are normal. It is also important to make sure there is no sign of pelvic infection. Simple tests will show the presence of an STI, vaginal infection, early cancer, or other conditions that may need to be treated. A blood sample may also be taken to make sure a woman is not anemic.

How Well IUDs Work

The chances of avoiding pregnancy when using an IUD are excellent. Only Norplant, sterilization, and Depo-Provera are more effective than IUDs in protecting against unplanned pregnancy. Fewer than 8 women in 1,000 who use a copper IUD will become pregnant during the first year of typical use. Only 6 will become pregnant with perfect use. Only 2 women in 100 who use an IUD with progestin will become pregnant during the first year of typical use. Only 15 out of 1,000 will become pregnant with perfect use. Even fewer pregnancies happen with continued use.

Intrauterine devices are more effective for women who have given birth than for those who have never been pregnant. The stretching of the uterus during pregnancy may make it less likely to reject an IUD.

A woman can increase her protection in two ways:

- by checking for the IUD string regularly and consulting with her practitioner if it is missing or is shorter or longer than at the time of insertion
- by using a condom, foam, or other barrier method when she is most likely to be fertile

Preparing for Insertion

An IUD is inserted into the uterus by a specially trained health professional.

To prepare for insertion, a woman will be asked a number of questions about her medical history and her lifestyle. The health care practitioner will want assurance, for example, that a woman has only one sex partner who has no other sex partners, because the IUD provides no protection against STIs. Being open and honest is extremely important because the IUD isn't suitable for all women.

THE PELVIC AND BIMANUAL EXAMINATIONS

After the medical history is recorded, a pelvic examination and bimanual examination are done. During the pelvic exam, the practitioner inserts an instrument called a speculum into the vagina. The speculum separates the vaginal walls enough so that the practitioner can see the vagina and cervix and make sure both are normal. After removing the speculum, the practitioner performs the bimanual exam by putting one or two fingers of one hand into the vagina. The other hand is placed on the abdomen. Then both hands are gently pressed together to check the size, shape, and position of the uterus and ovaries.

Often so much testing and discussion take place that a second appointment is necessary for the insertion itself. A woman should be sure to tell her clinician of any important changes that may have occurred between appointments—if she received a medical diagnosis or if she has a new sex partner. To avoid complications and remain healthy, a woman should keep her clinician informed.

SCHEDULING THE INSERTION

Finally, a woman must schedule the insertion. An IUD can be inserted at any time, but the most comfortable time may be during a menstrual period, when the cervix is softest. The menstrual fluid also provides lubrication during the insertion. It is also the time she is least likely to be pregnant. Another good time to have an IUD inserted is at midcycle because the cervix is naturally dilated during ovulation.

A woman planning to have an IUD inserted during a period or at midcycle should keep in mind that the first appointment may involve only testing and counseling. The insertion may have to take place at a future appointment.

Before insertion, a woman should discuss with her clinician

ways to spot possible side effects or other problems and should be sure to read the package insert that comes with the IUD before having one inserted.

The practitioner will also provide a woman with a consent form containing detailed information about the risks and benefits of the IUD she is considering. She needs to read, understand, and sign this form before the IUD is inserted.

When scheduling an insertion, a woman may want to arrange to have someone available to escort or drive her home afterward.

Insertion

Some practitioners instruct a woman who has scheduled an insertion to take an over-the-counter painkiller an hour or so before the procedure to lessen the cramps that insertion may cause. Because possible infection is a risk of IUD insertion, the woman may be given an antibiotic to protect against infection during and after insertion.

To insert the IUD, the clinician holds the vagina open with a speculum—as in a pelvic exam. An instrument called a tenaculum is attached to the cervix to steady the uterus. Then another, called a sound, may be inserted to measure the length of the cervical canal and uterus.

After the sound is withdrawn, a tube containing the IUD is inserted. The "wings" (T-bars) of the IUD bend back as they enter the uterus through the cervix. The IUD is pushed into place by a plunger in the tube. The wings spring open into the T-shape when the IUD is in the uterus.

Then the tube, plunger, tenaculum, and speculum are withdrawn, and the IUD is left in place with the filament hanging down through the cervix into the vagina. The clinician snips the string end to about an inch long. It can't be seen outside the vagina but is long enough to be felt by a finger inserted in the vagina.

During insertion there is some cramping pain. Some women feel a bit dizzy, and on rare occasions a woman may faint. The cramping eases with a little rest or pain medication. Many women feel nothing more than mild discomfort during insertion. Women with sensitive cervical tissue may have a local anesthetic injected around the cervix to reduce or prevent the pain.

At the time of insertion, a woman should note the type of IUD inserted and when it should be replaced. Otherwise, future clinicians will not be able to tell which IUD is being used and when it needs to be replaced.

Following insertion, a woman should plan to rest for the remainder of the day.

After Insertion

Some women adjust to their IUDs very quickly. Others may take several months to become entirely comfortable. Overall, women's level of satisfaction with IUDs is quite high. More than 60 percent of women who have IUDs inserted continue to use them for more than two years.

There may be some spotting between periods during the first few months, and the first few periods may last longer and the flow may be heavier.

Cramping or backache may occur for several days or weeks after insertion. Simple pain medication usually clears up cramping and discomfort. If bleeding or pain is severe and does not seem to be lessening, a woman should tell her clinician.

A woman should have a checkup following her first period after insertion. She should not wait longer than three months after insertion to make sure her IUD is still in place. A woman using an IUD should have checkups at least once a year to make sure everything is all right. This is usually done at the time of an annual Pap test.

Checking the IUD

Sometimes the uterus pushes out, or expels, an IUD. Expulsion is more common in women who have never been pregnant. It is more likely to happen during the first few months of use but may occur later.

An IUD can be expelled "silently" without the woman's knowledge. This is most likely to occur during a period. A woman should check her pads or tampons daily during menstruation to see if the IUD has fallen out. If expulsion occurs, a woman must check with her clinician and use another form of birth control—barrier methods such as male or female condoms, which are available over-the-counter—to protect against pregnancy.

The string attached to the IUD hangs from the uterus into the vagina, making it easy to check if the IUD is still in place. A woman should feel for the string regularly between periods. It is especially important to check every few days during the first few months after insertion.

To feel for the string, a woman should:

- Wash her hands, then either sit or squat.
- Put her index or middle finger into the vagina until it touches the cervix. The cervix will feel firm and somewhat rubbery, much like the tip of her nose.
- Feel for the string coming through the cervix. If the string is found, it means that the IUD is in place and working. However, if the string feels longer or shorter than before, it may be that the IUD has moved and needs to be repositioned by a health care professional. Another form of birth control should be used until it is repositioned.

Note: The string should never be pulled. Pulling might make the IUD move out of place or even come out. The IUD was carefully positioned during insertion; it shouldn't be disturbed.

Warnings That Something Is Wrong with an IUD

A woman should tell her clinician immediately if:

- She cannot find and feel the string.
- She thinks she might be pregnant.
- She has severe cramping or increasing pain in the lower abdomen that may be associated with feeling faint.
- She has pain or bleeding during sex.
- She has unexplained fever and/or chills.

- She has increased or bad-smelling vaginal discharge.
- She has a missed, late, or unusually light period.
- She has unexplained vaginal bleeding after the usual adjustment phase.

If the string of the IUD cannot be felt, the uterus may have pushed out the IUD without the woman knowing. It's also possible, although rare, that the IUD may have worked through the uterus into the abdomen, which could result in an internal injury. In either case, medical attention is required.

If the hard plastic bottom of the T of the IUD is felt against the cervix, it is not in the correct position and is not protecting the woman against pregnancy. She should tell her clinician immediately.

If a woman's periods last much longer than usual or the flow is much heavier than usual, she may become anemic. If that occurs, it may be necessary to have the IUD removed.

If a woman has severe pain or cramps in the abdomen, pain while having sex, an abnormal discharge, or a fever, she may have a pelvic infection. Medical treatment may be necessary. The infection may become worse if it is not treated promptly.

See page 125 for more information about the side effects and risks of IUD use.

Removal

Having an IUD removed or replaced is usually a simple matter. The clinician carefully tugs on the string ends at a certain angle, the IUD "wings" fold up, and the IUD slides through the opening of the cervix. Replacing the IUD with a new one can be done immediately after removal in most circumstances.

In rare cases, IUDs become embedded in the uterus and cannot be easily pulled free. In these cases, the cervix may have to be dilated and a surgical tool—forceps—may be used to free the IUD. A local anesthetic is used for such removals. In very rare cases, surgery becomes necessary. Women may have to be hospitalized for removals that require incision.

Most experts agree that the IUD should be removed for surgical procedures involving the cervix and uterus.

Warning: A woman should never try to remove her own IUD or ask a nonprofessional to do it for her. Serious damage could result.

Sexually Transmitted Infections and the IUD

Like the Pill, IUDs do not offer protection against STIs. An STI can permanently damage the reproductive system. The presence of an IUD during a sexually transmitted infection may cause complications. Women who may have been exposed to an STI should see their health care practitioners for an examination as soon as possible. Treatment may be necessary. The longer a woman waits, the greater her risk of developing a serious pelvic infection.

Latex or female condoms should be used during sexual intercourse with any partner who may have an STI.

Possible Problems and Side Effects While Using IUDs

Using an IUD offers less risk to a woman's life and health than pregnancy. However, there are some risks associated with any method of birth control. Serious problems connected with the use of the IUD are rare, but they do happen once in a while. Knowing what could happen is a woman's safeguard. The sooner she reports any problem to her clinician, the better her chances of avoiding serious complications.

HEAVY MENSTRUAL FLOW

Spotting between periods is common with IUD use. The Paragard Copper T 380A IUD may cause a 50 to 75 percent increase in menstrual flow. The Progestasert, on the other hand, may *decrease* the amount of bleeding—it may also prolong bleeding and increase the incidence of spotting.

MENSTRUAL CRAMPS

The Paragard Copper T 380A IUD generally increases menstrual cramping, while the Progestasert IUD may decrease painful periods.

EXPULSION

From 1.2 to 7.1 percent of IUDs are partially or completely expelled from the uterus in the first year, especially in the first few months after insertion. If the expulsion is "silent" and the woman does not notice it, she can easily become pregnant. One out of five expulsions goes unnoticed. One-third of the pregnancies that occur during IUD use are due to "silent expulsions." Expulsion is more likely among younger women and women who have never been pregnant.

UTERINE PUNCTURE

Rarely, in 1 out of 1,000 insertions, the uterus is accidentally punctured. This is usually discovered and corrected right away. If not, the IUD can "migrate" through the perforation into other parts of the pelvic area. Although this sounds painful, it usually isn't. Some women discover it has happened only after becoming pregnant. If an IUD migrates, surgery may be required to remove the IUD.

INFECTION

Even though the inserter is sterilized before use, it can push bacteria that are naturally found in the vagina into the uterus. A woman may also develop infections during the four months following insertion, when the cervix has not yet closed. After that time, if a woman and her partner have sex only with each other, there is no greater risk of infection than for a woman not using birth control.

A mild infection usually clears up with medical attention without having the IUD removed. Once in a while, more serious infection occurs, and the IUD may need to be removed. In rare cases, infection may cause sterility or the need to remove the reproductive organs. Left untreated, such an infection might become fatal.

INFERTILITY

Because untreated infections associated with IUDs may make it difficult or impossible to become pregnant, IUDs are generally not recommended for:

- young women who haven't had any children
- women who want more children
- women who have had trouble conceiving in the past

PREGNANCY

Most pregnancies happen to IUD users when their IUDs fall out without their knowing it. Rarely, a pregnancy happens with the IUD in place. If it does, there is a 50 percent greater chance of miscarriage. However, a woman may lessen the chance by 25 percent by having the IUD taken out as soon as possible. If a pregnancy continues with an IUD in the uterus, there is a risk to the woman of serious, perhaps life-threatening infection. There is less danger if the IUD is taken out. If the IUD cannot be located and removed, abortion may be considered.

Leaving an IUD in place during pregnancy also increases the risk of premature rupture of the membranes. This will cause premature loss of amniotic fluid and lead to a premature birth.

There is no association between IUD use and increased risk of congenital abnormalities. Although cases of fetal deformity in women with IUDs have been reported, the occurrence is no greater than for women who are not using birth control.

IUD users are less than half as likely to have an ectopic pregnancy—a fertilized egg that implants in a fallopian tube rather than the uterus—as women who use no contraceptive. But if pregnancy does occur during IUD use, there is an increased chance that the pregnancy may be ectopic. Ectopic pregnancies are more likely among Progestasert users—about half of the pregnancies that occur are ectopic. Surgery may be required to remove an ectopic pregnancy.

If a woman with an IUD suspects she is pregnant, she should contact her practitioner immediately. If she is pregnant and chooses to complete the pregnancy, she must have close medical supervision throughout her pregnancy.

Advantages of Using IUDs

- IUDs offer effective, long-term protection against pregnancy.
- IUDs are immediately effective and immediately reversible. Like users of other temporary methods, users of an IUD who want to become pregnant should have no problem doing so once it has been removed. Nine out of 10 women who want to conceive after having an IUD removed become pregnant within a year.
- IUDs offer great privacy because no one needs to know if a woman is using it. Occasionally, a man may feel the string of the IUD against his penis during intercourse. If so, a clinician can shorten the string.
- IUDs do not interfere with the sex act.
- IUDs do not interfere with a woman's hormonal balance—they do not change the copper or hormone levels in the body.
- IUDs can be used by women who are breast-feeding.
- The progestin in Progestasert helps reduce menstrual cramping and menstrual flow.
- With an IUD in place, a woman doesn't have to think about using birth control every day or every time she has sex.
- IUDs are less expensive than all other contraceptive methods, with the exception of continuous abstinence, withdrawal, outercourse, and periodic abstinence.

Where to Get IUDs and What They Cost

A woman can visit a local Planned Parenthood health center, health maintenance organization (HMO), or a private doctor. At this time in the United States, the variety of available IUDs is limited. A health care provider can be consulted for more information.

The exam, insertion, and follow-up visit range from $250 to $450. These services are priced according to income at some family

An IUD is often the best method of birth control for women who need a highly effective contraceptive but who cannot take the Pill or use other hormonal methods. Many women have chosen IUDs because they have serious cardiovascular diseases or diabetes and their health care practitioners have advised them not to take the Pill. Others who prefer IUDs to the Pill are women 35 or older who smoke. For such women, the IUD may have fewer side effects than the Pill. Older women would likely face increased risks to their lives and health if an unintended pregnancy occurred as a result of using a less effective method of birth control.

Disadvantages of Using IUDs

- There is increased risk of pelvic inflammatory disease and infertility for women who are at risk for sexually transmitted infections.
- Users commonly have increased menstrual cramping and prolonged and increased menstrual bleeding during the first few months of use.
- Users need to check for strings after every menstrual period.
- Insertion and removal must be done by a clinician.

planning clinics and are covered by Medicaid. Because this is a one-time cost, the longer the IUD is used, the more cost-effective it becomes. For example, the one-time insertion cost of $400 and up for a copper IUD that is used for 10 years works out to less per year than the cost of other forms of reversible birth control. On the other hand, the cost of a one-time insertion of the progestin-releasing IUD is less—about $200—but it can be used for only one year.

7

◆

Reversible Contraception— Hormonal Methods

- *Oral Contraception—The Pill*
- *DMPA Injections—The Shot*
- *Norplant—Implants*

In the 1930s, research was launched to find a hormonal treatment to alleviate menstrual pain. The search led to the invention of hormonal contraception. The first hormonal contraception was the Pill, which became available in 1960 and is now the most popular method of reversible contraception in the United States.

Thirty-one years later, American women were offered another hormonal option—implants inserted under the skin to provide five years of contraception—called Norplant. Two years after Norplant, DMPA (also called "the Shot"), an injectable method that lasts 12 weeks, became available.

Throughout history, millions of women dreamed that they might live their lives free from the burdens of unintended pregnancy. While there remains a very real need for more and better contraception, the introduction of hormonal contraception offered a great improvement in the lives of millions of women.

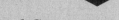

Oral Contraception—The Pill

"The Pill" is the common name for oral contraception. The two basic types, **combination pills** and **mini-pills,** both contain synthetic hormones similar to those produced by a woman's ovaries. Combination pills contain both estrogen and progestin, while mini-pills contain only progestin. Both types of pills require a medical examination, and a doctor's prescription.

Both kinds of pills are intended to prevent pregnancy, though they work in different ways. Combination pills *primarily* work by preventing the release of eggs from the woman's ovaries, an event

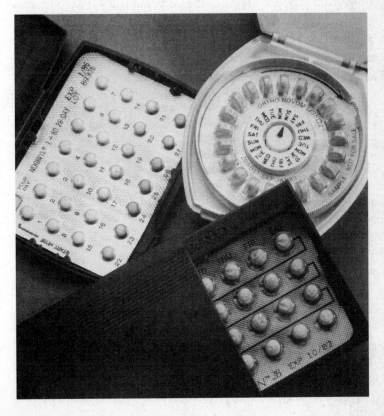

called ovulation. While mini-pills also can prevent ovulation, they *primarily* work by thickening the cervical mucus, creating a barrier that keeps sperm from joining with an egg. Combination pills also thicken cervical mucus. Both types of pills can also prevent fertilized eggs from implanting in the uterus (womb).

Today's low-dose combination pills contain 50 to 150 micrograms of progestin and 20 to 35 micrograms of estrogen. The mini-pill contains about 75 micrograms of progestin and no estrogen.

These dosages are only a fraction of those used in Enovid®, the first oral contraceptive approved by the U.S. Food and Drug Administration. The makers of the first pill wanted to be certain that it worked, so they used what are now know to be unnecessarily high levels of hormones. Enovid contained 10 milligrams (10,000 micrograms) of progestin and 150 micrograms of estrogen. It is no longer prescribed. Much of the current concern about the safety of the Pill stems from descriptions of side effects women experienced from the high dosages used in the Pill's early days.

Combination pills can be monophasic, biphasic, or triphasic. *Monophasic* means that the same dose of hormones is provided for each day of the menstrual cycle. Monophasic pills were the first type developed—Enovid was monophasic, for example.

Biphasic pills each contain a consistent level of estrogen but varying levels of progestin: For the first 10 days, the pills contain 0.5 milligram of progestin; for the next 11 days, they contain 1 milligram of progestin; and no pills at all are taken during the remainder of the menstrual cycle during which menstruation occurs. Biphasic pills are prescribed with much less frequency since the development of even lower-dose pills.

Triphasic pills have three phases of hormonal intensity that more closely replicate the normal monthly hormonal patterns of women. Tablets for each phase are a different color. Triphasic pills are preferred by some women and their health care practitioners because they retain the many health benefits of the Pill while reducing many side effects, including headache, nausea, depression, and unwanted hair growth.

Women Who Should Not Choose the Pill

Even with these advances, the Pill is not appropriate for all women who want to prevent unintended pregnancy. These include women who:

- smoke more than 15 cigarettes a day and are 35 or older
- smoke more than 15 cigarettes a day and are greatly overweight
- have had blood clots or inflammation of the veins
- have unexplained vaginal bleeding
- have had an abnormal growth or cancer of the breast or uterus.
- have a severe liver disease
- think they might be pregnant

Some women may be advised to take the Pill under close medical supervision because they have slightly high cholesterol, have slightly increased blood pressure, or have or have had diabetes—including diabetes associated with pregnancy. For them, the risk of pregnancy may be far greater than the risks associated with the Pill. Women with a history of depression or migraine headaches may not be able to take the Pill if it worsens the problem.

Getting the Right Pill

A woman must see a clinician to know whether she can take the Pill and what dosage is right for her. The clinician will take her medical history and give her other appropriate medical examinations.

If the Pill is right for her, a woman will likely be given a prescription for the lowest amount of hormone needed to protect her from unintended pregnancy. The clinician will adjust the prescription if the woman continues to experience side effects after a few months. Women should be sure to have checkups at least once a year. A prescription may need to be changed as a woman's health needs change. A woman should see her clinician as soon as possible if any problem develops.

A woman should remember to tell any other clinician she may see that she takes the Pill. This is particularly important if she's having a blood test for cholesterol, blood sugar levels, or thyroid disease.

Remember that pills are specifically prescribed for individual women—pills should never be shared or borrowed.

How Well the Pill Works

The Pill is one of the most effective reversible methods of birth control. Of 100 women who use the Pill, only 5 will become pregnant during the first year with typical use.

Combination pills are somewhat more effective than mini-pills. Only one out of 1,000 women who use combination pills will become pregnant during the first year with perfect use. Five out of 1,000 who use mini-pills will become pregnant with perfect use.

Myths about Failure Rates

Many women hear claims that the Pill is not very effective. They may not know that most of the "failures" attributed to the Pill occur because many women who say they are taking the Pill do not take it consistently or correctly. Here are the facts. A recent survey of women who take the Pill found that:

- Only 28 percent of women take the Pill correctly.
- Only 42 percent take the Pill every day.
- At least 16 percent have pills left at the end of the month.
- About 25 percent stop using the Pill before a year has passed and do not use another method.
- About 17 percent do not take the pills in the right order.
- About 33 percent of teen women missed a pill in a three-month period.

Women who take combination pills consistently and correctly—without fail—have a one-in-a-thousand chance of becoming pregnant.

How the Pill Is Affected by Some Other Medications

Some Medications That May Reduce the Effectiveness of the Pill

Type	Examples
antibiotics	rifampin (Rifadin®, Rimactane®)
anticonvulsants	carbamazepine (Tegretol®) phenytoin (Dilantin®) primidone (Mysoline®) barbiturates (Phenobarbital® and others)
antifungals	griseofulvin (Fulvicin®, Grisactin®, Gris-PEG®)

Some Medications That May Be Less Effective When Used with the Pill

Type	Examples
analgesics	acetaminophen (Pamprin®, Tylenol®, Paracetamol®, aspirin-free Excedrin®, and others)
anticoagulants	warfarin (Coumadin®, Panwarfin®)
antihypertensives	methyldopa (Aldoclor®, Aldomet®)
hypoglycemics	Diabinese®, Orinase®, Tolbutamide®, Tolinase®

Some Medications Whose Effects May Be Exaggerated When Used with the Pill

Type	Examples
antidepressants	amitriptyline (Elavil®, Endep®) imipramine (Tofranil®, Norpramin®, and others)
beta-blockers	Corgard®, Inderal®, Lopressor®, Tenormin®
bronchodilators	theophylline (Primatene®, Theo-Dur®, Marax®, Bronkotabs®, Quibron Tedral®, and others)
tranquilizers	benzodiazepam (Valium®, Ativan®, Librium®, Serax®, Tranxene®, Xanax®, and others)

In addition, large doses of vitamin C can exaggerate the effects of the hormones in the Pill. Women who use the Pill should take no more than 100 milligrams of supplemental vitamin C per day. A health care practitioner or pharmacist should be consulted about any medications taken while on the Pill.

Certain medicines, including the antibiotic rifampin and drugs used to control seizures, may make the Pill less effective. Vomiting and diarrhea also may keep the Pill from working. A clinician can be asked for advice if there is concern that vomiting or diarrhea may have affected the effectiveness of the pill. Until a woman is sure she is protected against pregnancy, she should use an additional method of birth control.

It is very important to remember that the Pill does not protect against sexually transmitted infections (STIs). A latex or female condom should be used along with the Pill for protection against STIs.

How to Use the Pill

Staying on schedule is very important. Correct and consistent use of the Pill increases a woman's protection against pregnancy. This method of birth control works best for women who are able to take the Pill at the same time every day without fail.

It is very important not to skip pills, even if there is spotting or bleeding between periods or if vaginal intercourse does not occur very often.

Pills come in monthly series, each in a separate pack. A whole series must be taken in the right order for the Pill to work.

Combination pills usually come in 28-day packs and are taken without interruption. The first 21 pills in the pack of combination pills are called "active"—they contain hormones that prevent pregnancy. The last seven pills in the pack of combination pills are called "reminder" pills. They are inactive pills that do not contain hormones. They are taken during the fourth week, when menstruation usually occurs, to help a woman stay in the habit of taking a pill on a regular basis.

Combination pills also come in 21-day packs. All 21 of the pills are "active." The pills are taken for three weeks. No pills are taken during the fourth week, when menstruation usually occurs. A new pack of pills is started seven days after the last pack is completed.

Mini-pills come only in 28-day packs. All mini-pills are "active." Some women will have an increased number of days of light bleeding. Others will have no menstruation.

A woman should be sure to follow the instructions on the package.

What to Do If You Forget

If you forget ONE active combination pill:	Take it as soon as you remember. Take the next pill at the usual time. (This means you may take two pills in one day.) Finish that series and start the next pack on time.
If you forget TWO active combination pills in a row in the first two weeks:	Take two pills on the day you remember. Then take two pills on the next day. Take one pill every day until the pack is finished. Use a backup method for seven days after the pills are skipped. Call your clinician if you do not start your period.
If you forget TWO active combination pills in a row in the third week—or you forget THREE or more active combination pills in a row during the first three weeks:	**Sunday starters:** Take one *active* pill every day until the next Sunday. Throw away the rest of the pack and start a new pack the same day (Sunday). Also use a backup method for seven days after the pills are skipped. You may not have your period this month, but this is expected. Call your clinician if you do not get your period two months in a row. **First-day starters:** Throw away the rest of the pack. Start a new pack the same day. Use a backup method for seven days after the pills are skipped. You may not have your period this month, but this is expected. Call your clinician if you do not have a period two months in a row.
If you forget ANY of the seven reminder pills in the fourth week:	Throw away the pills you missed. Take one of the remaining reminder pills each day until the pack is empty. Start the next pack on time.
If you forget EVEN ONE mini-pill:	Take it as soon as you remember. Take the next pill at the usual time. (This means you may take two pills in one day.) Continue to take the rest of the pack on schedule. Use a backup method of birth control for the rest of the month. Start the next pack on time.
If you are still not sure about the pills you have missed:	Use a backup method any time you have vaginal intercourse. Take one active pill each day until you can talk with your clinician.

Missing pills can cause spotting or light bleeding—even if you make up the missed pills. You also may feel a little sick to your stomach when you take two pills to make up for missed pills.

Myths about Taking a "Rest" from the Pill

One of the many myths about the Pill is that women should occasionally take a "rest" from taking the Pill. However, this is unnecessary because:
- There are no medical benefits.
- Taking a rest from the Pill can lead to unintended pregnancy.
- Discontinuing and restarting the Pill may cause another round of unpleasant side effects associated with the first few months of pill use.
- Women who discontinue the Pill sacrifice some of the noncontraceptive benefits of the Pill.

The only reason to take a rest from the Pill is to plan a pregnancy.

The clinician will explain how to use the pill pack—either the 28-day or 21-day pack. Taking the Pill at the same time each day makes it more effective. It also helps a woman remember to stay on schedule. A woman should pick a time of day that will be easy to remember. For example, the pill pack can be kept next to the toothbrush.

The clinician will advise a woman to start the pill on a Sunday or on the first day of her period. If she is a "Sunday starter," she should take the first active pill of the first pack on the Sunday after her period starts—even if she is still bleeding. If her period begins on Sunday, the pack should be started that same day. Pills are then taken daily according to the schedule provided in the pack—one every day for 28-day packs or one every day for 21-day packs followed by seven days off.

Another method of birth control should be used during vaginal intercourse during the first week after beginning the Pill—anytime from the Sunday the first pack is started until the next Sunday. Good backup methods include male or female condoms, a diaphragm, or a cervical cap. Protection will begin after seven days and continues as long as the Pill is taken on schedule.

Myths about Weight Gain and the Pill

Many women believe that they will "get fat" if they take the Pill. While the hormones in the Pill may cause some appetite changes that result in weight loss or gain, "getting fat" usually results from lack of exercise and/or overeating. Many studies have been done that prove that, on average, taking the Pill does not change a woman's weight.

Pill users with 28-day packs should start the next pack the day after finishing the previous pack—regardless of when menstruation takes place. Pill users with 21-day packs should start the next pack seven days after finishing the previous pack.

If a woman starts the Pill on the first day of her period, she should take the first active pill of the first pack during the first 24 hours of her period. "First-day starters" have no need to use a back-up method of birth control. Protection against pregnancy begins immediately and continues as long as the Pill is taken on schedule.

Side Effects of Using the Pill

As with all drugs, there may be some undesirable side effects for some women taking the Pill. However, the Pill is much safer than pregnancy and childbirth for healthy women—except among smokers age 35 and older. Because the dose of hormones in the Pill has been decreased and refined over the years since it was first introduced, the side effects of the Pill today are minimal.

Some side effects that usually clear up after two or three months of use include:

- bleeding between periods
- weight gain or loss
- breast tenderness
- nausea—rarely, vomiting
- depression
- decreased sex drive

Advantages of Using the Pill

- The Pill is an extremely effective method of contraception.
- The Pill is simple and convenient to use.
- Using the Pill does not interrupt intercourse.
- The mini-pill can be used while breast-feeding. The combination pill can be used while breast-feeding six weeks after delivery.
- The Pill offers contraceptive protection within seven days. It is immediately effective if started by Day 7 of the menstrual cycle.
- The Pill is easily reversible.

Noncontraceptive Benefits of Using the Pill

The Pill offers many health benefits, including some protection against:

- infections of the fallopian tubes (pelvic inflammatory disease, or PID), which commonly lead to infertility
- ectopic pregnancy
- benign breast tumors
- ovarian cysts
- cancer of the ovaries
- cancer of the lining of the uterus
- menstrual irregularity and menstrual cramps
- iron-deficiency anemia

The Pill increases the presence of cervical ectopia, in which the surface of the cervix remains sheathed in mucus-secreting cells and does not develop a covering of protective cells. Ectopia makes the cervix more vulnerable to chlamydial infections, but there is no evidence that the Pill increases a woman's risk for PID.

Some women inherit a predisposition that may metabolize the hormones in the Pill to produce side effects such as acne, body and

- rheumatoid arthritis
- acne
- menopausal vaginal dryness and painful intercourse
- osteoporosis (thinning of the bones)

In fact, protection against developing cancer of the ovary or the lining of the uterus can last up to 15 years after stopping the Pill. Protection against endometrial cancer increases with each year of use—women who use the Pill for eight years reduce their risk of getting endometrial cancer by up to 80 percent.

The possibility that the Pill offers protection against uterine fibroids has yet to be proven conclusively.

Disadvantages of Using the Pill

- Effectiveness is seriously jeopardized if a woman does not take the Pill every day—forgetfulness increases failure.
- The Pill offers no protection against sexually transmitted infections.
- The Pill has unpleasant side effects for some women.
- The Pill poses serious health risks for some women— especially those with a tendency for increased blood clotting.
- Return to fertility can be delayed up to three months.

facial hair growth, male-pattern scalp hair loss, and vaginal dryness. These side effects often clear up in three months for most women. Nausea and vomiting often can be reduced or eliminated by taking the Pill with the evening meal or at bedtime. (A woman should not stop taking the Pill if she feels sick to her stomach.) Irregular spotting and bleeding happen more frequently with mini-pills than with combination pills.

Myths about Safety and the Pill

More than 60 percent of women mistakenly believe that oral contraception is more risky than or as risky as childbirth. In fact, childbearing carries twice the risk of death as does the use of the Pill.

Once in a while, menstruation is irregular or absent for as long as six months after stopping the Pill. This generally occurs if periods were irregular before starting the Pill.

Rare Serious Problems

The most serious problem associated with the Pill is the possibility of blood clots in the legs, lungs, heart, or brain.

Women on the Pill who undergo major surgery seem to have a greater chance of having blood clots. Blood clots in the legs occur with increased frequency for women and men who have one or both legs immobilized or who are confined to their beds. It is important to stop taking the Pill about four weeks before a scheduled major operation. A woman should not start again while recuperating or while a leg or arm is in a cast.

Rarely, high blood pressure may develop in women who take the Pill. The rise usually is slight. But it may worsen over time.

Myths about Cancer and the Pill

Most experts agree that taking the Pill does not increase the overall risk of developing breast cancer—no matter how long a woman takes the Pill—even if she has a close relative with breast cancer. Allegations that the Pill is associated with cancer of the liver and cervical cancer have yet to be proven.

Stopping the Pill almost always brings blood pressure back to normal. A woman should be sure to have her blood pressure checked after her first three months on the Pill and monitored at least once a year after that.

Very rarely, liver tumors, gallstones, and jaundice (yellowing of the skin or eyes) occur in women who take the Pill. Though very rare, liver tumors occur most often in women who have used the Pill five years or more. They usually subside when the Pill is stopped. Occasionally, surgery is required. Most pill-related cases of jaundice and gallstones occur within the first year of use.

In extremely rare cases, heart attack or stroke associated with Pill use can threaten life. The chances increase with age among women who have had blood vessel disorders or who have other health problems. These problems include diabetes, high cholesterol, high blood pressure, significant obesity, and, most of all, smoking. Pill-related risks of heart attack or stroke go away once the Pill is stopped. Heavy smoking (more than 15 cigarettes a day) is the greatest risk factor related to taking the Pill. Women over 35 must not smoke and take the Pill.

If the Pill is stopped to resolve these or other such problems, another method of birth control must be used to prevent pregnancy. More detailed information about the use and risks of the Pill is provided in an insert included with each pill pack.

Myths about Heart Attack, Stroke, and Blood Clots and the Pill

There is no increase in the risk of heart attack or stroke among healthy women who use the Pill and who do not smoke. There is a small increase in the risk of blood clots in the legs and arms. The increase is from 5 to 20 cases of blood clots among 100,000 women per year to 15 to 20 cases of blood clots among 100,000 women per year.

EARLY WARNING SIGNS

Rare serious problems associated with taking the Pill usually have warning signs. If one occurs, a woman should report it to her clinician as soon as possible. These warning signs include:

- sudden or constant pain or redness and swelling in the leg
- sudden shortness of breath or spitting up blood
- sudden pain in the abdomen, chest, or arm
- severe headache
- sudden blurred or double vision or loss of vision in one eye
- worsening depression
- yellowing of the skin or eyes (jaundice)
- weakness of arm, leg, or face on one side of the body

Smoking or the Pill?

Smoking is one of American women's greatest health risks.

- Women who smoke die nearly 16 years earlier than nonsmokers.
- Smokers are much more likely to develop progressive lung disease and lung cancer—the number-one cause of cancer death for American women.
- Smoking increases the risk of cervical cancer.
- Smokers have twice as much heart disease—those who smoke more than a pack a day have three times the rate of heart disease as nonsmokers.
- Smoking is also associated with cancers of the mouth, throat, pancreas, and bladder.

In addition, babies of smoking mothers are more likely to be born prematurely, have low birthweight, or be disabled or die in infancy. Smoking also harms the health of "secondary smokers"—those who breathe in other people's smoke—especially children.

Pregnancy and the Pill

There is a very slight chance that pregnancy will occur even if the Pill is taken regularly, especially if there is vomiting or diarrhea or certain medications have been used.

A missed period usually does not mean a pregnancy, especially if no pills have been skipped. But it is important to see a clinician if a second period is missed. It is unlikely that taking the Pill during early pregnancy will increase the risk of defects in the fetus. However, the likelihood of ectopic pregnancy is greater if pregnancy occurs while taking the mini-pill.

If a woman wants to become pregnant, she should simply stop taking the Pill. If she wants to plan her pregnancy, she should use

Taking the Pill and smoking are a deadly mix. A Pill user who smokes more than 15 cigarettes a day takes very serious health risks. The older the woman and the more she smokes, the greater the danger. The risk of death is much higher for women over 35 who smoke and use the Pill than it is for nonsmokers over 35.

A woman over 35 who takes the Pill and smokes must give up one or the other. This is especially true if she has diabetes, high blood pressure, or elevated cholesterol, because these conditions further increase the risk of heart attack or stroke.

A woman must choose another form of birth control if she cannot stop smoking. Quitting smoking isn't easy, but it may be easier than having an unintended pregnancy as a result of using a less effective method of birth control.

Other health benefits are gained by becoming smoke-free. Within two years of quitting, a large proportion of the increased risk of heart disease disappears. Ten to 15 years after quitting, an ex-smoker's chance of early death from lung cancer drops to about the same as someone who never smoked at all.

> ### *Myths about Birth Defects and the Pill*
>
> The Pill does not cause birth defects or affect the health of future children—even if a woman becomes pregnant while taking the Pill.

another form of birth control until her period becomes regular. This usually takes one to three months.

After childbirth, a clinician can help a woman decide when to take the Pill again. Mini-pills will not affect breast milk during nursing. Combination pills may reduce the amount and quality of milk in the first six weeks of breast-feeding. Also, the milk will contain traces of the Pill's hormones. It is unlikely that these hormones will have any effect on a child.

Where to Get the Pill and What It Costs

A prescription can be obtained from Planned Parenthood health centers, health maintenance organizations (HMOs), or a private health care practitioner such as a doctor. Pills may be purchased at a drugstore or at the Planned Parenthood health center from which they are prescribed.

The cost of an examination by a private doctor may range from $50 to $125. Family planning clinics usually charge according to income. Pills vary in price depending on the type and brand. A prescription filled at a drugstore costs about $15 to $25 a month. The cost usually is less at a health center and is covered by Medicaid. Some private insurers cover the cost of contraception, when its use is authorized by a health care professional.

DMPA Injections—The Shot

DMPA, also called "the Shot," is a progestin—a synthetic hormone similar to progesterone, one of the hormones that regulates the menstrual cycle. The full name of the hormone is depot medroxypro-

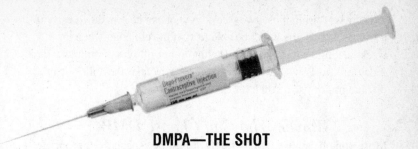

DMPA—THE SHOT

gesterone acetate (DMPA). The brand name is Depo-Provera®. An injection of DMPA in the buttock or arm can prevent pregnancy for 12 weeks. DMPA keeps the ovaries from releasing eggs and also thickens cervical mucus to keep sperm from joining eggs. DMPA also thins the lining of the uterus to prevent implantation in the unlikely event that an egg is fertilized.

Before prescribing DMPA, a clinician will take a family and medical history and perform other appropriate medical examinations.

The standard dose of DMPA is 150 milligrams. DMPA is injected into the arm or buttock and may leave a temporary bruise at the injection site. Follow-up shots are required every three months, so it is important for a woman to choose a clinician who will be available during hours that are convenient.

A shot is needed every 12 weeks for as long as a woman wants to prevent pregnancy. The medication actually lasts slightly longer than 12 weeks, so there is a two-week grace period if the next appointment needs to be postponed. However, effectiveness begins

DMPA and Breast Cancer

The U.S. Food and Drug Administration (FDA) has reviewed the speculation and allegations that DMPA is associated with breast cancer and has found that there is no increased risk of breast cancer among women who use DMPA.

to decrease during those two weeks. A shot can be scheduled early if a woman knows she won't be able to visit the clinician when the 12-week deadline comes around. Having to put off an appointment for a day or two is not as risky as forgetting to take the Pill, put in a diaphragm, or use a condom.

Women Who Can Choose DMPA

Most women can use DMPA safely. It may be especially appropriate for women who:

- want very effective long-lasting contraception
- want long-term birth spacing
- cannot take estrogen
- can accept changes in the pattern of their menstrual bleeding
- are unable to use barrier methods routinely or take a daily pill

WOMEN ABLE TO USE DMPA UNDER SPECIAL MEDICAL SUPERVISION

It may not be advisable for a woman to use DMPA without special clinical supervision if she has:

- concerns about gaining weight
- diabetes
- migraine headaches
- major depression
- high cholesterol or blood pressure
- recent history of liver disease (such as hepatitis) or abnormal results on liver function tests

Women Who Should Not Choose DMPA

A woman should not choose DMPA if she:

- is or might be pregnant
- cannot put up with irregular bleeding or loss of her period
- wants to become pregnant within 18 months of having her last injection
- has unexplained vaginal bleeding

- has a severe liver dysfunction or disease or a history of growths of the liver
- has had a heart attack or stroke
- has ever had breast cancer
- has Cushing's syndrome—an adrenal dysfunction—and is being treated with aminogluethamide (Cytadren®)
- recently had blood clots in the eyes, legs, or lungs

How Well DMPA Works

DMPA is one of the most effective reversible methods of birth control. Of every 1,000 women who use it, only 3 will become pregnant during the first year.

Protection is immediate if the injection is given during the first five days of the period. Otherwise, an additional method of contraception should be used for the first two weeks. Protection lasts for 12 weeks.

DMPA injections provide no protection against sexually transmitted infections, including HIV.

DMPA, Bone Thinning, and Teens

There is some concern that the use of DMPA may lead to the bone thinning condition osteoporosis. This concern is largely based on a small 1991 study done in New Zealand that suggested that DMPA may slightly decrease bone density. The findings remain inconclusive.

Studies are under way to determine whether DMPA may actually contribute to osteoporosis. Until the results of those studies become available, many clinicians have decided to refrain from prescribing DMPA for girls between ages 12 and 14 because they do not want to risk interfering with the important bone-building process that goes on during this period of a girl's life.

Side Effects of DMPA

Irregular bleeding is the most common side effect for women using DMPA. Periods become fewer and lighter for most women. Fifty percent of women who use DMPA will stop having their periods after one year of use; 80 percent will have no periods after five years of use. It may take a year for periods to begin again after a woman stops using DMPA. Other women will have longer and heavier periods. Some may have more light spotting and/or breakthrough bleeding.

Irregular bleeding is likely to subside with time, but women who experience irregular bleeding while using DMPA may want to consider alleviating the condition by taking a short course of estrogen therapy, one or two cycles of the Pill, or ibuprofen.

For about two months after the first injection, about one in four

Advantages of Using DMPA

- DMPA is a very private method—no one can tell if a woman is using it.
- DMPA is one of the safest and most effective methods.
- DMPA prevents pregnancy for 12 weeks.
- DMPA has few method-related health risks.
- DMPA doesn't need to be taken daily or put in place before having vaginal intercourse.
- DMPA doesn't require surgery or insertion.
- DMPA can be used by some women who cannot take estrogen.
- DMPA can be used while breast-feeding. It does not affect the quality of milk, although there are some indications it may increase the volume of milk produced.

Noncontraceptive Benefits of Using DMPA

- DMPA reduces menstrual cramps and anemia.
- DMPA protects against endometrial and ovarian cancers.
- DMPA protects against some causes of pelvic inflammatory disease.

women taking DMPA has side effects that mimic the symptoms of pregnancy, such as nausea and sore breasts.

Less common side effects include:
- increased appetite and weight gain
- headache
- nervousness
- dizziness
- depression
- skin rashes or spotty darkening of skin
- hair loss
- increased facial or body hair
- vaginal dryness
- increased or decreased sex drive

- DMPA protects against ectopic pregnancy.
- DMPA may alleviate the symptoms of sickle-cell anemia and endometriosis.

Disadvantages of Using DMPA

- Side effects cannot be neutralized or reversed for 14 weeks after injection. Irregular bleeding and other side effects may even continue for up to eight months until DMPA is cleared from the body.
- DMPA involves getting a shot every 12 weeks.
- DMPA offers no protection against sexually transmitted infections.
- The effects of using DMPA cannot be reversed immediately.
- It may take as long as 18 months for a woman to become pregnant after she stops using DMPA.
- Some women and their partners may find unpredictable breakthrough bleeding to be unpleasant during sexual activity.

Warning Signs

Some side effects of DMPA use can actually lead to or be signs of more serious problems. Heavy vaginal bleeding can lead to significant anemia. Feelings of sadness may signal the onset of depression. Sudden and severe abdominal pain may be the symptoms of an ectopic pregnancy, in the unlikely event that DMPA failed to prevent pregnancy.

A woman should tell her clinician immediately if she has:

- vaginal bleeding that lasts longer and is much heavier than her usual period
- severe headaches
- major depression
- frequent urination
- yellowing of the skin or eyes

DMPA and Pregnancy

Another area of concern is the possibility of harmful effects on the development of a fetus inadvertently exposed to DMPA. While a single study suggested that early-pregnancy exposure to DMPA may increase the likelihood of premature birth, experts question whether these results are valid. As an extra precaution, clinicians who prescribe DMPA should ensure before giving the drug that a woman is not pregnant. DMPA appears to have no adverse effects on infants exposed to the drug while breast-feeding.

Where to Get DMPA and What It Costs

DMPA is available from Planned Parenthood health centers, health maintenance organizations (HMOs), or private medical practitioners. The cost of an examination ranges from about $35 to $125. The injection costs about $50. Subsequent visits may cost $20 to $40, plus the injection. The total cost for each year of use will be between $215 and $545. At health centers, costs may be less, based on income. All costs are covered by Medicaid. Some private insurers cover the cost of contraception, when its use is authorized by a health care professional.

If a woman is more than two weeks late for her shot, a pregnancy test may be required before she receives the next injection. Pregnancy tests cost up to $20.

Norplant—Implants

Norplant implants are thin, flexible plastic rods. Six are inserted under the skin of the upper arm to provide the most effective reversible contraception. The soft capsules are about the size of a cardboard matchstick. They are made of Silastic®, a silicone material that has been used safely since the 1950s for prosthetic replacements, such as heart valves. Each capsule contains powdered crystals of the hormone levonorgestrel, which is a progestin—a synthetic version of the progesterone made by a woman's ovaries.

The capsules continually release a small amount of the progestin. The progestin keeps the ovaries from releasing eggs and also thickens the cervical mucus, keeping sperm from joining with an egg. Some researchers believe that the progestin may also thin the lining of the uterus, preventing a fertilized egg from implanting in the uterus and starting a pregnancy.

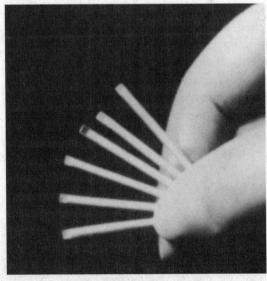

NORPLANT IMPLANTS

Protection against pregnancy begins within 24 hours if the insertion is done during the first seven days of the menstrual cycle. Protection lasts for five years.

Women Who Can Choose Norplant

These include women who:

- want continuous, long-acting birth control
- do not want to take a pill daily or put a contraceptive in place before having vaginal intercourse
- do not want to use a method that contains estrogen
- can put up with some irregular bleeding and spotting

Women Able to Use Norplant under Special Medical Supervision

Women who use Norplant should be checked regularly by their clinicians if they have:

- increasingly severe, constant headaches
- diabetes
- high cholesterol or blood pressure
- heart disease
- severe liver dysfunction or disease
- seizures that require medication
- serious depression
- conditions that may be aggravated by fluid retention

Women Who Should Not Choose Norplant

These include women who:

- are pregnant
- cannot put up with irregular bleeding
- have unexplained vaginal bleeding
- have ever had breast cancer
- are breast-feeding in the first six weeks after delivery
- have a history of growths of the liver

- have a history of a certain kind of high blood pressure—idiopathic intracranial hypertension
- have a certain kind of brain tumor—meningioma
- are sensitive to the ingredients in Norplant

Where to Get Norplant

A woman must see a clinician to find out if she can use Norplant. The clinician will take a medical history and perform other appropriate medical examinations.

How Well Norplant Works

Norplant is one of the most effective reversible methods of birth control available in the United States. It becomes effective within 24 hours of insertion and protects against pregnancy for five years. Of every 1,000 women who use Norplant for five years, 5 will become pregnant—this is only one per year. Norplant is actually slightly more effective than sterilization, but the contraceptive effect disappears a few hours after the implants are removed.

Certain medicines, such as those used to control seizures, may make Norplant less effective. A woman should ask her clinician for advice whenever she is given new medication—especially for treatment of seizures or tuberculosis. An additional method of birth control should be used if the woman is unsure that the medication is affecting the contraceptive effectiveness of the implants.

How Norplant Is Used

Insertion

Norplant usually is inserted during the first seven days after the start of the menstrual period. This is to be certain the woman is not pregnant. Another form of birth control should be used until the insertion is done. Norplant can be inserted immediately after an abortion or when an old set of implants is removed. It can be inserted at any time of the month if the Pill or an IUD is being used. It also can be inserted immediately after childbirth in women who are not breast-feeding. If a woman is breast-feeding, she can use Norplant six weeks after childbirth.

If Norplant is appropriate for the woman, the clinician will wash the skin with an antiseptic and numb a small area of the upper arm with an anesthetic. The clinician will make one small cut—usually less than one-quarter inch in length. Six capsules will be inserted under the skin of the arm used least. All six capsules are needed to prevent pregnancy. They will be placed in a fan-shaped pattern

Advantages of Using Norplant

- Norplant is the most effective method of reversible contraception.
- Norplant provides protection against unintended pregnancy for five years.
- Norplant can be used by some women who cannot take estrogen.
- Norplant has no serious method-related health risks.
- Norplant is generally "carefree." There are no supplies to purchase, pills to remember, or devices to insert.

Disadvantages of Using Norplant

- Norplant requires minor surgery to insert and remove.
- Norplant provides no protection against sexually transmitted infections.
- Women are dependent on their clinicians for insertion and removal. The method cannot be reversed by women themselves.
- Norplant can be a relatively expensive method if removal takes place within three years.

under the skin. Insertion takes about 10 minutes. While the insertion may be unpleasant, it is painless except for the needle prick of the anesthetic.

A small bandage will be applied to the spot, but stitches are not needed. The bandage should be left in place for three days and kept away from water. It may be wrapped in protective gauze. If the gauze is too tight, there may be numbness in the arms and fingers.

It's common to experience some itching, tenderness, and swelling for a few days after the bandage comes off. If symptoms persist longer or if the arm hurts or looks red, a woman should call her health care provider. Relatively few people develop an infection, but it is always possible when the skin is broken for any reason.

If a woman's skin is very thin or her arm is very muscular, the capsules may look like protruding veins. Otherwise they're invisible.

Heavy lifting should be avoided for about a week after insertion. A temporary bruise may appear at the insertion site, and there may be some discomfort for a few days.

A woman will also be advised to make a follow-up visit within the first three months after insertion to make sure that she is not having any problems. It is best to have follow-up visits once a year after that. A woman should remember to tell any health care provider she sees that she is using Norplant.

Removal

Norplant must be removed five years after insertion. It can be removed anytime earlier, if desired. Removal is important because hormones may continue to be released in amounts sufficient enough to create menstrual irregularities but insufficient enough to prevent pregnancy.

For removal, the clinician will numb the area with an anesthetic. One small cut will be made to remove all six of the implants. Several incisions may be needed because the implants are more difficult to locate in some women. Removal takes longer than insertion—usually from 15 to 20 minutes—and more than one visit may be required. New implants may be inserted at this time. A woman who is susceptible to scarring may have raised scars after removal.

Why Do Women Ask to Have the Implants Removed?

Irregular bleeding is the reason that 9 percent of the women who use Norplant ask to have it removed. About 5 percent report headaches or other symptoms as the chief reason. Another 5 percent want to have a baby.

In the last several years, uncomfortable side effects and painful removals have triggered a round of lawsuits. Many women, concerned by the controversy, have asked to have their implants removed. In response, Wyeth-Ayerst, the manufacturer, has created a nonprofit organization called the Norplant Foundation to issue certificates for low-income women who want their implants removed but can't afford the fees. The foundation's toll-free number is 800-736-6775. The manufacturer has also issued a patient acknowledgment form that has been incorporated into the product's labeling, to be used at the time of prescription. This form allows consumers to acknowledge receipt of information and gives them the opportunity for thorough discussion regarding Norplant prior to insertion. Wyeth-Ayerst also has a product information hotline from which consumers can obtain information about Norplant and the names of providers who are experienced in the insertion and removal of it. The toll-free number is 800-934-5556.

Unless the woman wants to become pregnant, she should use another form of birth control if Norplant is removed.

For insertion and removal, it is important to choose a health care practitioner who is experienced in the insertion and removal of Norplant. If the implants are inserted too deeply, they may be more difficult to remove. If they have been in place longer than five years, they may become more embedded, making removal more difficult.

Side Effects Associated with Using Norplant

As with all medicines, there may be side effects for some women using Norplant. The most common side effect of Norplant is irregular bleeding. About 70 percent of women using Norplant experience menstrual changes during the first year of use. Irregular intervals between periods occur for 55 percent of the women who use Norplant, and irregular bleeding or spotting between periods occurs among 45 percent. Some women may have a longer or heavier menstrual flow, while others may have no menstrual bleeding for months at a time. Some 25 percent have no period during the first 90 days; another 10 percent have no periods for three to four months at a time.

Bleeding usually becomes more regular after 9 to 12 months. Usually there is less blood loss with Norplant than with a normal period. A woman thinking about using Norplant must be able to tolerate unpredictable menstrual periods. A small number of women experience irregular bleeding throughout the five years.

There are other side effects for some women. These include side effects similar to those reported by some women who use the Pill. They include:

- possible scarring at insertion and removal
- headache
- change in appetite
- weight gain or loss
- depression
- dizziness
- nervousness
- sore breasts
- nausea
- changes in sex drive
- decreased vaginal lubrication
- acne
- gain or loss of hair on face or body
- discolored skin over the implants

- raised (keloid) scars at the insertion site (more likely in women of color)
- enlarged ovaries or fallopian tubes
- increased chance of ectopic pregnancy in the unlikely event that pregnancy occurs
- ovarian cysts (rare)

Rare Serious Problems

Norplant works very much like the Pill. It is not yet known if some of the rare problems that occur with the Pill may also occur with the use of Norplant. Until more studies show otherwise, Norplant users (especially those who smoke) may be at slightly increased risk for heart attacks and strokes. Blood clots and inflammation of the veins are also possible side effects.

Smoking while using the Pill greatly increases the risks of heart attack and stroke in women who are over 35 years old. It is not yet known if this happens with Norplant. For now, women using Norplant are advised to stop smoking.

WARNING SIGNS

Serious problems are very rare. Usually there are warning signs:
- vaginal bleeding that is *much* heavier than a normal period
- delayed menstruation after a long period of regular cycles
- arm pain
- severe lower abdominal pain, especially if it is on one side
- severe headaches and/or blurred vision
- pus or bleeding at the implant site after insertion or removal
- one of the implants that seems to be coming out
- nerve pain while moving the arm or hand after the insertion site has healed

A woman should report any warning signs to her clinician as soon as possible.

Pregnancy and Norplant

Although very rare, pregnancy can occur while a woman is using Norplant. If pregnancy occurs, Norplant should be removed. If a woman wants to become pregnant, she should have the implants removed. Her ability to become pregnant will be the same as it was before using Norplant.

ECTOPIC PREGNANCY

Women who use Norplant have fewer ectopic pregnancies than women who use no birth control. However, in the rare case when Norplant fails, there is a greater chance that the pregnancy will be ectopic—that is, the fertilized egg will implant outside the uterus.

Ectopic pregnancies are life-threatening conditions and must be treated. They can be removed with surgery, or they can be treated medicinally. Warning signs include a late period and severe lower abdominal pain. If these occur, a woman should see her health care provider immediately.

Where to Get Norplant and What It Costs

Norplant is available from Planned Parenthood health centers, HMOs, or private medical practitioners. Norplant costs between $500 and $750 for the medical exam, the implants, and the insertion. This amounts to a little more than $100 a year over a five-year period. The fee for removing Norplant ranges from $100 to $200. All costs are covered by Medicaid. Clinics may charge less. Some private insurers cover the cost of contraception, when its use is authorized by a health care professional.

Chapter

8

◆

Emergency Contraception

Emergency contraception is designed to prevent pregnancy after unprotected vaginal intercourse takes place. It is also called post-coital or "morning-after" contraception.

At some time in their lives, most women are faced with the fear that they might have an unintended and unacceptable pregnancy. In fact, the average woman spends 75 to 80 percent of her fertile years trying to avoid pregnancy. During that time she may forget to use a contraceptive, her contraceptive may fail, or she may be coerced into having unprotected vaginal intercourse.

Women in most developed countries have had access to emergency contraception for several decades. Until recently in the United States, the use of emergency contraception was limited to rape crisis centers, college health clinics, and family planning health centers. Most American women have been unaware of emergency contraception or how to get it.

Researchers estimate that emergency contraception could prevent more than half of all the unintended pregnancies and abortions that take place in the United States every year. They point out that lower rates of unintended pregnancy in other developed nations may be due to the greater access to emergency contraception for women in those countries. Many family planning professionals have referred to emergency contraception as America's "best-kept secret."

Unfortunately, most American women think that the only option they have after unprotected intercourse is to wait and see. Emergency contraception can alleviate the stress of this wait and the decisions that may follow.

While most physicians know about emergency contraception, most don't prescribe or talk about it unless a woman asks. Most American women, however, don't know enough about emergency contraception to ask for it.

What Is Emergency Contraception?

Emergency contraception is provided in two ways: emergency hormonal contraception (in the form of birth control pills) or emergency insertion of an intrauterine device (IUD).

Emergency contraception prevents pregnancy by preventing fertilization (the union of sperm with an egg) or implantation (the attachment of a fertilized egg to the wall, or lining, of the uterus).

Emergency Hormonal Contraception

Emergency hormonal contraception is a sequence of two doses of certain oral contraceptives (see Chapter 7, "Reversible Contraception—Hormonal Methods"). The most commonly used "morning-after pills" are combination pills, which contain estrogen and progestin—synthetic hormones like the ones produced by a woman's body. Combination pills used for emergency contraception are taken in two doses (see chart on page 168), 12 hours apart, started within 72 hours of unprotected intercourse. Progestin-only pills—called mini-pills—may also be used for emergency contraception. They are taken in two doses of 20 pills, 12 hours apart, started within 48 hours of unprotected intercourse. Progestin-only pills are most appropriate for women who cannot take estrogen.

Any woman who can take the Pill can use morning-after pills—if she is not pregnant. To be certain, the woman's health care provider may order a pregnancy test. Some practitioners will also suggest a

Is Emergency Contraception Abortion?

Gynecologists and most other women's health care providers agree that pregnancy begins when the fertilized egg implants itself in the lining of the uterus. The hormones that support pregnancy—the ones detected by pregnancy tests—are not present until implantation has taken place. More than 85 percent of obstetrician/gynecologists who refuse to perform abortions for personal or religious reasons have said that they would prescribe emergency contraception for their patients.

gynecological exam unless the woman has had one recently. Others may require a follow-up appointment.

Take-home kits of emergency contraception pills are also available from family planning and women's health centers. A woman who keeps an emergency hormonal contraception kit at home can take the medication immediately following unprotected intercourse without having to wait to see her clinician. A woman who does not have pills and who cannot get to a clinic may be able to get a physician to call in a prescription to her pharmacy. Health care providers are much more likely to do so for women whose medical histories are known to them. Women who request emergency contraception pills—to use immediately or to take home for emergency situations—should review their medical histories with their clinicians before receiving the packs.

A woman should not use the morning-after pills if she:
- is pregnant
- has missed her period or it is late
- is allergic to the medication

Emergency IUD Insertion

Emergency IUD insertion can be done by a clinician within five to seven days of unprotected intercourse. The insertion of an IUD into the uterus can prevent the preembryo from being implanted there.

The Paragard Copper T 380A is the only IUD used for emergency contraception in the United States. It can be left in place for up to 10 years to provide long-term contraception (see Chapter 6, "Reversible Contraception—Intrauterine Devices"). Or if she prefers, the IUD can be removed after the woman's next menstrual period, when it is certain that she is not pregnant.

IUD insertion for emergency contraception isn't recommended for women who are at risk for sexually transmitted infections. These include women who have more than one sex partner or whose sex partner has more than one partner, women who have recently started a new sexual relationship, and women who have been raped.

The side effects, advantages, and disadvantages of using IUDs for emergency contraception are the same as those associated with using IUDs for ongoing contraception (see page 125).

How Well Emergency Contraception Works

Emergency hormonal contraception. A woman's risk of pregnancy varies from day to day during her menstrual cycle. Emergency hormonal contraception initiated within 72 hours of unprotected

---

Why a Woman Might Need Emergency Contraception

- Her partner's condom broke or slipped off, and he ejaculated inside her vagina.
- She was forced into having unprotected vaginal intercourse.
- Her diaphragm or cervical cap slipped out of place, and her partner ejaculated inside her vagina.
- Her partner didn't pull out in time.
- She miscalculated her "safe" days for periodic abstinence or fertility awareness methods.
- She wasn't using any birth control.
- She forgot to take the Pill more than two days in a row.

intercourse reduces the risk of pregnancy by at least 75 percent. If, for example, a woman's risk of pregnancy is 8 percent at the time, hormonal contraception will reduce her risk to 2 percent or less. If, on the other hand, her risk of pregnancy is 24 percent at the time, hormonal contraception will reduce that risk to 8 percent or less.

Emergency IUD insertion. Insertion within five to seven days of unprotected intercourse reduces the risk of pregnancy by 99.9 percent.

It is important to remember that emergency contraception pills help prevent a pregnancy from only one act of unprotected intercourse. They do not continue to prevent pregnancy during the rest of the cycle. Other methods of birth control must be used. This means that if a pre-embryo has already implanted in the lining of the uterus and pregnancy has begun, emergency contraception will not end the pregnancy.

Emergency contraception may also not prevent an ectopic pregnancy. An ectopic pregnancy is one that develops outside the uterus and is a medical emergency that is fatal unless treated. Signs of ectopic pregnancy include:

- severe pain on one or both sides of the lower abdomen
- abdominal pain and spotting, especially after a missed menstrual period or a very light one
- faintness or dizziness

Babies born to women who used "morning-after pills" without knowing they were pregnant have not had higher rates of birth defects than other babies. But there is still some concern that a fetus may be damaged if emergency contraception pills are used during pregnancy.

Emergency contraception will not protect against sexually transmitted infections.

Preparing to Use Emergency Contraception

If you request emergency contraception, your health care provider may want to know the following:

- Do you have any symptoms of pregnancy, such as nausea, swollen breasts, or fatigue?

- When did you have your last period and was it abnormal in any way?
- What are your normal, shortest, and longest menstrual cycles?
- What is the date of your expected ovulation during the current cycle?
- Have you had other unprotected intercourse during your present menstrual cycle?
- How many hours has it been since unprotected intercourse took place?
- What do you usually use for contraception?
- What method of contraception would you like to use after using emergency contraception?

You may be asked to sign a consent form stating that you understand how emergency contraception works and its potential risks.

Note: Be sure you have the emergency phone number for the health center or clinician who provides your emergency contraception.

How to Use Emergency Contraception Pills

Several types of oral contraceptives can be used for emergency contraception. You must use only one type of pill and use it for all doses. (See chart on page 168.) Combination pills, which contain estrogen and progestin, are more effective than mini-pills, which contain only progestin. Progestin-only pills may be more appropriate for women who cannot take estrogen.

USING COMBINATION PILLS FOR EMERGENCY CONTRACEPTION

If you take your emergency hormonal contraception from a regular 28-pill pack of combination pills, you can use any of the first 21 pills for emergency contraception—the last seven pills in the pack are only reminder pills that contain no hormones. If you use Triphasil® or Tri-Levlen®, the first 21 pills are in three different colors, and you must use only the yellow ones.

Dosages of Combination Pills for Emergency Contraception

Brand Name	Pills in First Dose	Pills in Second Dose
Ovral®	2	2
Lo/Ovral®	4	4
Nordette®	4	4
Levlen®	4	4
Triphasil (yellow only)	4	4
Tri-Levlen (yellow only)	4	4

First dose: Swallow the pills in the first dose as soon as possible and no later than 72 hours—three days—after having unprotected intercourse. Because nausea is a possible side effect, you may want to eat a snack of soda crackers or drink a glass of milk shortly before taking each dose to reduce the risk of vomiting.

Your clinician may prescribe antinausea medication or suggest one that you can buy over-the-counter, such as Dramamine®. The side effects of antinausea medication may include lightheadedness, dizziness, or a spacey feeling. Be sure to follow the precaution listed on the package insert.

Second dose: Swallow the second dose 12 hours after taking the first dose. If vomiting occurred after the first dose, be sure to use an antinausea medication 30 minutes before taking the second dose. Or you may want to take the second dose vaginally. If so, the pill must be deeply inserted into the vagina; otherwise, it is more likely to fall out. If you vomit the second dose, do not take any extra pills—it is unlikely that they will reduce the risk of pregnancy any further. It is likely that they will increase your risk of nausea.

USING PROGESTIN-ONLY PILLS FOR EMERGENCY CONTRACEPTION

If your clinician prescribes mini-pills for emergency contraception: Swallow 20 pills of Ovrette® within 48 hours of unprotected intercourse, and then swallow another 20 pills 12 hours later. Women who use mini-pills experience less nausea.

KNOWING WHAT TO EXPECT AFTER TAKING EMERGENCY CONTRACEPTION PILLS

After you take emergency contraception pills:

- Your next period may be earlier or later than usual.
- Your flow may be heavier, lighter, or more spotty than usual.
- If you see other health care providers before you menstruate, remember to tell them that you have taken emergency hormonal contraception.
- Schedule a follow-up visit with your clinician in three weeks if you do not menstruate or if you have other symptoms of pregnancy.
- Plan to use another method of contraception if you have vaginal intercourse before your period.

Emergency contraception is meant for emergencies only. It is not as effective as many other forms of reversible contraception, including Norplant, Depo-Provera, and continuous use of an IUD or the Pill. If you have sex with more than one partner, or your partner does, use male or female condoms for protection against sexually transmitted infections (STIs), including HIV.

If you suspect you are pregnant any time after you take the "morning-after pills," you should have a pregnancy test and pelvic examination. The signs of pregnancy include:

- a missed period or unusually light period
- nausea and vomiting
- breast tenderness or enlargement
- fatigue

Remember: Emergency contraception may not prevent ectopic pregnancy. If you think you may have an ectopic pregnancy and cannot reach your health care provider, go to a hospital emergency room.

Side Effects Associated with the Use of Emergency Contraception Pills

- Nausea, usually mild, is experienced by 50 percent of women who use emergency hormonal contraception.
- Up to one out of three women experiences vomiting.
- Cramping is likely.
- Breast tenderness, irregular bleeding, fluid retention, and headaches may also occur.

If you use emergency hormonal contraception frequently, your periods may become quite irregular and unpredictable.

Where to Get Emergency Contraception and What It Costs

If you have unprotected intercourse during a time when you think you might become pregnant, contact your health care provider immediately. Emergency contraception is available from Planned Parenthood health centers, other family planning and public health clinics, private doctors, and hospital emergency rooms (unless a hospital is affiliated with a religion that opposes the use of birth control). It is expected as we go to press that the U. S. Food and Drug Administration will soon approve the packaging and sale of emergency hormonal contraception packets.

To contact the Planned Parenthood health center nearest you, call 800-230-PLAN.

Bridging the Gap Communications, Inc., an Atlanta publisher, has produced a small paperback, *Emergency Contraception: The Nation's Best-Kept Secret*. It can be ordered by calling 800-721-6990. Updated regularly, the book contains a state-by-state, city-by-city list of clinics and health care providers who are willing to provide emergency contraception.

You can get the names, addresses, and phone numbers of three emergency contraception providers nearest you by calling the toll-

Advantages of Using Emergency Contraception

- Emergency contraception is highly effective.
- Emergency contraception reduces the need for abortion.
- Emergency hormonal contraception is easy to use. Intrauterine devices used for emergency contraception can be used as an ongoing method of contraception.
- Side effects of emergency contraception are short-lived.
- Emergency contraception can alleviate some of the anxiety following rape or other coerced sexual intercourse.

Disadvantages of Using Emergency Contraception

- Emergency contraception cannot be used by all women.
- Emergency contraception pills have unpleasant side effects for half the women who use them.
- Emergency contraception may not protect against ectopic pregnancy.
- Emergency IUD insertion is usually inappropriate in circumstances that include risk for STIs—rape, coercion, or other situations in which the sexual health of partners is unknown.
- Getting a prescription for emergency contraception pills within three days of unprotected intercourse may be difficult in some instances.

free **emergency contraception hotline: 888-NOT-2-LATE.** The list, which now contains about 1,600 U.S. providers, is continually updated. The fully automated, 24-hour number provides several choices, including a number to press for recorded information about emergency contraception.

The complete updated list can also be found on the World Wide Web at the following Internet address:

http://opr.princeton.edu/ec/ec.html

Emergency contraception kits cost $8 to $15 at clinics and other health centers. A visit to a health care provider's office or clinic for counseling and a prescription may cost as little as $35 at a clinic or as much as $150 at a private physician's office. The pregnancy test at a clinic may cost an additional $10 to $20. For a full pack of the pills themselves, the cost is about $20 for a pack of combination pills and about $50 for two packages of mini-pills. The total costs vary widely, from a low of $8 to a high of $245, depending on the medical services that are required.

The ParaGard Copper T 380A IUD costs about $400 for the exam, the IUD, and insertion. It lasts for 10 years, however, so the cost of the IUD—if left in place—works out to only $40 a year.

Medicaid and some private insurers cover the cost of emergency contraception, when its use is authorized by a health care professional.

Chapter

9

◆

Permanent Contraception— Sterilization

• *Vasectomy—Sterilization for Men*
• *Tubal Sterilization—Sterilization for Women*

Voluntary sterilization is the most popular method of birth control in America. More than a million women and men choose to have the procedures every year. Sterilization is surgical birth control—it is intended to be permanent, and it is not easily reversed. **Vasectomy** is the surgical operation for men. It blocks the tubes that carry sperm. **Tubal sterilization** is the surgical operation for women. It blocks the fallopian tubes where eggs are fertilized by sperm. Vasectomy is more effective and less expensive and complicated than tubal sterilization.

Usually, people choose sterilization when they have completed their families and have had all the children they want. Most of them are over 30 and married. Some women and men, however, choose sterilization in their earlier reproductive years because they know they never want to have children. Others choose sterilization because

173

they have a hereditary condition that they do not want to pass on to another generation. Still others choose sterilization when the woman is chronically ill or physically disabled in a way that would make pregnancy very difficult or dangerous.

Couples often choose voluntary sterilization after they have had to deal with a pregnancy "scare" or an abortion. Because sterilization procedures are nearly 100 percent effective, couples who do choose sterilization have very little concern about the chance of unintended pregnancy for the rest of their lives. Because sterilization is intended to be permanent, it is inappropriate for young women or men who, as they mature, may change their minds about having children.

◆

Vasectomy—Sterilization for Men

Vasectomy is permanent birth control for men. It is a surgical operation that is intended to cause sterility. About 500,000 men in the United States choose vasectomy every year. It is chosen by men who have completed their families or by men who want no children. These men want birth control that will last for as long as their partners are fertile. They prefer vasectomy because most reversible methods are less reliable, are sometimes inconvenient, and may have unpleasant side effects for the women in their lives.

Vasectomy is a simple operation. It makes a man sterile by keeping sperm out of his ejaculate, the fluid that spurts from the penis during sex. Pregnancy can happen if a sperm joins with a woman's egg.

Sperm are produced in the testicles. They pass through two tubes called the vasa deferentia to other glands and mix with seminal fluids to form semen. Vasectomy blocks each vas deferens and keeps sperm out of the seminal fluid. The sperm are absorbed by the body instead of being ejaculated. Without sperm, a man's ejaculate cannot cause pregnancy.

Vasectomy does not affect masculinity, and it does not affect a man's ability to get hard or stay hard. The same is true for the sex organs, sexuality, and sexual pleasure. No glands or organs are removed or altered. Hormones and sperm continue being produced. The ejaculate will look just like it always did, and there will be about as much of it as before.

Mentally competent men can legally choose vasectomy in all 50 states. No one who is mentally competent can be forced to have the operation. Welfare benefits cannot be denied to men who refuse vasectomy. Attempts to do so are against federal law.

Policies, practices, and access to vasectomy vary with individual doctors, hospitals, and health centers. Vasectomy may be difficult to arrange under some circumstances—for instance, if a man is young, single, or childless.

Men do not need to have the consent of their wives or other partners, but discussion with them is very important. Waiting periods before the operation are sometimes required to allow more time for thought before the procedure takes place. For federally funded vasectomies, men must:

- be at least 21 years old
- observe a 30-day waiting period after signing a statement of informed consent
- be free of the influence of alcohol or other drugs at the time of consent
- reapply if the procedure is postponed for more than 180 days

How Well Vasectomy Works

Vasectomy is the most effective form of birth control for sexually active men. A man and his partner will need no other contraceptive after a successful vasectomy. Sterilization must be regarded as permanent, even though it may be reversible in some cases. Any decision to have no biological children in the future must be firm. A man must be absolutely sure he will never change his mind or regret his choice—no matter how his life changes.

Vasectomy is nearly 100 percent effective. Of 1,000 women

whose partners have vasectomies, only 1 will become pregnant in the first year. Risk is increased if they have sex too soon after the procedure.

Vasectomy is not immediately effective. Sperm remains in the system beyond the blocked tubes. A man must use other birth control until the sperm are used up. This usually takes from 15 to 20 ejaculations. A simple test—semen analysis—shows when there is no more sperm in the seminal fluid. The follow-up exam for semen analysis will be scheduled at the time of the operation. If repeated semen analyses reveal continued presence of sperm, a man may have to consider having a second vasectomy. This is rare. Very rarely, tubes grow back together again and pregnancy may occur. This happens in 1 out of 1,000 cases in the first year.

Providing a semen sample can be done in the laboratory or at home, although samples provided at home must be delivered to the laboratory within a few hours. Most men masturbate in order to provide a sample. Special condoms, also used for sperm donation, are available to collect the sperm during masturbation or intercourse. Test results may be available in three days.

Vasectomy offers no protection against sexually transmitted infections. Sexually transmitted infections can be carried in ejaculate whether or not it contains sperm.

Antibodies to sperm develop in 50 percent of men who have vasectomies. Normally, antibodies protect the body against viruses and bacteria. Sperm antibodies will not affect general health, but they will kill sperm and may lessen the chance of restoring fertility if the vasectomy is reversed.

Men Who May Want to Consider Vasectomy

Men may consider vasectomy for many reasons, including the following:

- They want to enjoy having sex without causing pregnancy.
- They don't want to have a child in the future.
- Their partners agree that their family is complete and no more children are wanted.

- They or their partners have concerns about the side effects of other methods.
- Other methods of birth control are unacceptable to them.
- They don't want to pass on a hereditary illness or disability.
- They want to spare their partners the surgery and expense of tubal sterilization—sterilization for women is more complicated and costly.
- Their partner's health would be threatened by a future pregnancy.
- They are comfortable with their masculinity and know that a vasectomy won't affect their sex life.

Men Who Should Not Consider Vasectomy

Vasectomy should not be considered by men under the following conditions:

- They are in their teens or early 20s.
- They may want to have a child in the future.
- They are being pressured by a partner, friends, or family. *The man* must want the operation.
- They want to solve a temporary problem. Marital or sexual problems, short-term mental or physical illnesses, financial worries, being out of work, and other circumstances that may change are not good reasons for vasectomy.
- They have not considered possible changes in their lives, such as divorce, remarriage, or death of children.
- They have not discussed vasectomy fully with their partner.
- They plan to bank sperm in case they change their mind. (Sperm banks collect, freeze, and thaw sperm for alternative insemination.) Some men's sperm does not survive freezing. In addition, after six months, frozen sperm may begin to lose the ability to fertilize an egg.
- They are under too much stress to make such an important life-long decision.
- They remain concerned that vasectomy may affect their masculinity or their ability to maintain an erection.
- They are counting on reversal if they change their mind.

Alternatives to Vasectomy

A man should consider all other methods of contraception before he chooses vasectomy. The Pill, Norplant, Depo-Provera, and IUDs are more than 95 percent effective. Most women can use them with little risk of serious complications. Other methods that have few or no side effects are diaphragms, cervical caps, male and female condoms, periodic abstinence, fertility awareness methods, and contraceptive foams, jellies, and suppositories.

A man's partner may want to consider sterilization. There are new sterilization procedures for women that reduce the cost, recovery time, and extent of the surgery. But vasectomy is still simpler, less costly, and less risky than the procedures available to women. In all cases, the results must be considered permanent. Both partners need to think carefully about what sterilization will mean for both of them—and their futures.

Getting a Vasectomy

FIRST STEP—THE MEDICAL EXAM

Before deciding whether a man is a good candidate for a vasectomy, he and his doctor will discuss his medical history. He will also have a physical examination, including laboratory tests of samples of blood and urine.

Many men are sterile without knowing it. If a man has had mumps during adulthood or if he has any other reason to think he may be sterile, he should be sure to discuss the possibility with his doctor. It may be appropriate for him to have a semen analysis to discover whether a vasectomy is necessary.

The doctor will consider a man's psychological as well as his physical health to determine if he is a good candidate for a vasectomy. Often the first step is counseling by the surgeon or someone else who is knowledgeable about the subject, such as a nurse or social worker. The counselor will make sure the man understands what a vasectomy involves and that he has considered other contraceptive options. Talking with other men who have had vasectomies may be helpful. If a man doesn't have a friend he can ask, the doctor may provide the name of someone who may be helpful.

A man may be asked to consider how he would feel if, after vasectomy, he lost his current partner and took another who wanted a child. What if his existing child or children died?

Once a man has decided to proceed, he will be asked to sign consent forms attesting to the fact that he understands all aspects of what will and may happen before, during, and after a vasectomy.

SECOND STEP—PERSONAL PREPARATIONS

In preparation for a vasectomy, a man should:

- Get his shopping done. He will need an athletic supporter or snug Jockey®-type briefs to wear after the surgery. Either will keep the gauze dressings in place and keep the weight of the scrotum from pulling on the wound. He will need to wear the strap for the first 48 hours and during the day for the following week. He may want to have two straps so that he can wash one while he wears the other. An ice pack and a box of gauze pads may come in handy, too. An ice pack may be soothing after surgery, and there may be further bleeding.
- Arrange for someone to drive him home after surgery.
- Arrange to take some time off work after the operation. A man should expect to be sore enough to appreciate a couple of days off his feet at home. He may want to incorporate a weekend into the days he takes off—Friday is a popular day for vasectomies.
- Plan to have someone else be with the kids. A man should be sure someone is around to give a hand—at least for the first 24 hours after returning home. Even if the kids are away, he may want an adult around to make things more comfortable.
- Fill any prescription for painkillers the doctor thinks he may need. He should be sure he has the medication before the procedure. He will not want to go pick it up afterward.
- Avoid taking aspirin or any medications containing aspirin during the week before the surgery. Aspirin thins the blood and interferes with clotting. If a man ordinarily takes aspirin or any

other blood thinner, such as warfarin (Coumadin®), for a medical condition, he should consult his doctor.

- Avoid drinking alcohol or taking any other drugs on the night before surgery, unless the doctor has approved doing so. A man may get permission to take a mild sedative on the day of the procedure to stay calm. This may help relieve stress that can tighten the muscles and increase pain.

- Ask the doctor for a telephone number that may be called 24 hours a day after surgery in case of an emergency.

- Avoid eating or drinking anything except a little water for at least eight hours before surgery.

- Contact the physician if a cold, fever, flu symptoms, or any other infection develops—especially a genital rash, boil, pimple, or other skin condition—shortly before his appointment. He may have to reschedule.

- Cancel the surgery if there are any last-minute doubts. A man should not go through with the surgery just because the arrangements have been made.

- Wash the penis and scrotum carefully while bathing for a few days before surgery—the cleaner they are, the more resistant to infection they'll be.

- Shower or bathe on the morning of the surgery and wash the scrotum with extra care, possibly with an antibacterial soap such as pHisoHex® or Betadine®. The man will not be able to shower or bathe for a couple of days after the vasectomy. He may also be asked to shave the scrotum in the shower so the hair gets washed away. The hair above the penis can be left in place.

- Wear loose and comfortable pants and underwear. He should not forget to take along an athletic supporter or a clean pair of briefs for after the surgery.

THIRD STEP—THE PROCEDURE

There are two types of procedures, the conventional vasectomy and the newer procedure, known as a microvasectomy or no-scalpel vasectomy. They differ in the way the doctor gets to the tubes.

- **Conventional Vasectomy.** Conventional vasectomy is performed with the use of a scalpel. The doctor numbs the scrotum by injecting a local anesthetic. Two cuts are made in the skin. The tubes are lifted, one at a time, through the incisions. They are cut and blocked to prevent sperm from getting into the man's ejaculate. The tubes are eased back into the scrotum, and the doctor stitches the incisions closed. Conventional vasectomy takes about 20 minutes.

- **No-Scalpel Vasectomy.** The newer "microvasectomy"—no-scalpel method—is done without making incisions in the scrotum. The scrotum is numbed with an injection of a local anesthetic. The doctor feels for the tubes under the skin and uses a small clamp to hold them in place. A tiny puncture in the scrotum is made with a special instrument. The instrument gently stretches the opening so the tubes can be reached. The tubes are cut and blocked with same procedures used in conventional vasectomy. No-scalpel vasectomy usually takes about 10 minutes.

There are several advantages of having a no-scalpel vasectomy instead of a conventional vasectomy.
- There are no incisions.
- There are no stitches.
- The procedure takes less time.
- The recovery is faster.
- There is less chance of bleeding and other complications.
- There is less discomfort after the operation.
- The no-scalpel method is just as effective as the conventional method.

Whatever method is used, the doctor will remove a segment of each tube. The segments are sent to a laboratory for examination to be positive that each tube that was cut was a vas deferens and not a ligament or blood vessel. This precaution ensures that if in the rare circumstance an error was made in the procedure, it will be detected.

Closing Off Each Vas Deferens

There are several techniques doctors use to close the ends of the tubes to prevent the tubes from spontaneously reconnecting. This spontaneous reconnection—called recanalization—is rare but accounts for a significant proportion of failures associated with vasectomy.

- **Tying (ligation).** Once the ends have been cut, the doctor folds them back and ties off each one with surgical thread. This method is the most widely used in the United States but has the highest risk of recanalization.
- **Metal clips.** The cut ends are closed off with metal clips. Damage to the tubes caused by the clips reduces the risk of recanalization and the chances of reversal.
- **Electrocautery.** A very thin wire is inserted into the open ends of each cut vas. A high-frequency electric current quickly coagulates the inner tissue, sealing the end with a scar. Electrocautery is the most effective way to reduce the risk of recanalization and the chances of reversal.

However the ends are closed, the sheath that covers the vas is pulled over the cut end and sewn closed.

In a variation called an open-ended vasectomy, the surgeon closes only one end of each vas. The tube leading from the testis is left open to relieve pressure of potential sperm build-up in the epididymis (the tube that carries the sperm from the testes to the vas deferens).

Closing Up

After the vasa deferentia have been cut or sealed, the ends of the tubes are eased back into the scrotum. For a very small incision or puncture, the doctor may use no sutures. The skin will heal in less than a day and the incision will become invisible in two weeks. For other incisions, the doctor may use either self-absorbing sutures that dissolve in about a week or nonabsorbable sutures that must be removed. If the doctor uses nonabsorbable sutures, a man should expect to return to the office in five to seven days to have them removed.

Sterile gauze will be applied to the incision or puncture site. A man will rest for up to half an hour and will be asked to urinate to check for complications. He can go home as soon as he feels up to it.

FOURTH STEP—RECUPERATING

A man may be given a prescription for a painkiller if he has not received one already. However, for most men, strong painkillers like codeine are usually unnecessary. Nonaspirin painkillers such as Tylenol® every four to six hours may be all that is needed. If pain relief is needed three days after surgery, the doctor may give a man permission to take straight aspirin.

At home, an ice pack should be put on the scrotum for at least four hours to reduce swelling, bleeding, and pain. There will probably be a dull ache in the groin area when the anesthesia wears off an hour or two after the surgery. Within a couple of days, a man should feel fine.

As with any surgery, mild bleeding can occur for a few days after the procedure. There may be a little ooze of blood on his bandage for a day or two. A man should contact his doctor if he needs to change his bandages more than a couple of times a day.

After two days, he can take a bath or shower.

FIFTH STEP—RESUMING NORMAL ACTIVITIES

The doctor will let a man know when he can exercise or play sports. Waiting two or three weeks should be sufficient. If his job involves heavy physical labor, especially lifting heavy objects, he should discuss the situation with his doctor in advance. A letter from his doctor may help him get reassigned to lighter work for a short time. In any case, he should be careful not to overdo it.

A man can resume having intercourse two or three days after surgery or whenever he feels ready after that. He should expect some discomfort at first if he does have intercourse, since the vasa deferentia, which will be sore after the operation, normally contract during ejaculation. His discomfort will diminish as he heals.

Risks Associated with Vasectomy

Vasectomy is low-risk surgery. Complications can occur with any kind of surgery. Major complications with vasectomy are rare and are usually associated with infection. Other potential problems include:

- Bruises caused by bleeding into the skin during surgery. These will clear up by themselves.
- Swellings containing blood, called hematomas. These occur in fewer than 3 out of 100 cases. They usually clear up by themselves or with bed rest or ice packs. Surgical drainage is rarely needed.
- Swellings containing fluid, called hydroceles, and tenderness near the testicles. This occurs in less than 1 out of 100 cases and usually clears up in about a week. Applying heat and wearing an athletic supporter help. Surgical drainage is rarely needed.
- A small lump, called a granuloma, caused by sperm leaking from the tubes. A granuloma appears under the skin near the site of the operation in about 18 out of 100 cases. Sperm granulomas are usually painless and clear up by themselves. Surgical treatment is sometimes required if a granuloma persists and causes discomfort.

Vasectomy and Prostate Cancer

Study results have been inconsistent and weak. Those that show an association between vasectomy and prostate cancer demonstrate only very small differences between men who have had vasectomies and men who have not. Researchers have concluded that there is no biological relationship between vasectomy and prostate cancer. However, all men between 50 and 70 years old should be screened for prostate cancer every year—whether or not they have had vasectomies. Men who have had vasectomies should be screened no differently from those who have not had vasectomies.

Psychological Side Effects

It is very important for men who consider voluntary sterilization to receive thorough and unbiased counseling. A man who has thoroughly explored his options and feels comfortable with his decision will most likely feel good about choosing vasectomy for the rest of his life.

Regret occurs among 5 to 10 percent of the men who choose vasectomy. Depending on their emotional status before the operation, their regret may be associated to varying degrees with depression, a sense of guilt, lowered self-esteem, or a diminished conviction in their masculinity.

Rarely, men lose some sexual desire. More rarely, men lose the ability to become erect. Most often, such losses are also related to their emotional status before the operation.

- Mild infections. These occur in up to 7 out of 100 cases. Rarely, an abscess may develop. Treatment with antibiotics is successful.
- Recanalization. Very rarely, the cut ends of a vas deferens grow back together. This most often happens within four months of the operation and may allow pregnancy to happen.
- Adhesions or fistulas. In rare instances, the tissues may bind to form areas of thick scar tissue. These may require surgical correction.
- Decreased sexual desire or inability to become erect. This occurs in 4 out of 1,000 cases. The most likely cause is emotional—there is no physical cause for sexual dysfunction associated with vasectomy.

A man should contact his clinician if he has any sign of serious problems:
- fever over 100.4°F
- blood or pus oozing from the site of the incision
- excessive pain or swelling

Where to Get a Vasectomy and What It Costs

A vasectomy may be arranged through a family health care provider, health maintenance organization, local hospital, local public health department, or Planned Parenthood health center. An appointment with the nearest Planned Parenthood health center may be scheduled by calling toll-free, 800-230-PLAN.

Advantages of Having a Vasectomy

- Vasectomy provides permanent, highly effective contraception.
- Vasectomy is inexpensive in the long term.
- Vasectomy is a simple surgery that can be done under local anesthesia.
- Vasectomy has no proven, significant, long-term, medical side effects.
- Vasectomy offers great privacy.
- Vasectomy does not rely on partner compliance.
- Vasectomy does not interrupt sexual activity.
- Vasectomy is one of the few methods that allows a man to take responsibility for contraception.

Disadvantages of Having a Vasectomy

- Vasectomy is a surgical procedure.
- Men who choose vasectomy will experience short-term pain and discomfort.
- Reversal is expensive and cannot be guaranteed.
- Vasectomy may cause infertility despite successful reversal.
- Vasectomy offers no protection against sexually transmitted infections.
- Vasectomy is not immediately effective.
- Vasectomy is expensive in the short term.
- Five to 10 percent of men have regrets about choosing the operation.

Information about vasectomies is also available from AVSC (Access to Voluntary and Safe Contraception International), 79 Madison Ave., 7th Floor, New York, NY 10016; 212-561-8000.

Vasectomy is usually performed in a clinic or doctor's office. Hospitalization may be necessary for men with serious heart disease or any other medical condition that makes it necessary for them to be monitored continuously throughout the surgery.

Fees for vasectomy range between $240 and $1,000 for an interview, counseling, examination, operation, and follow-up sperm count. (Sterilization for women costs up to four times as much.) Some clinics and doctors use a sliding scale according to income. A man who is considering the procedure should also know whether his health insurance will cover most or all costs.

Blue Cross and Blue Shield and some private health insurance policies may pay some or most of the cost. In about 35 states, Medicaid pays but puts some restrictions on patient eligibility. A man should check with his local department of social services to see if he is covered.

Some insurance companies may not cover vasectomies done in a hospital. Check with your insurer. If a man needs the benefits of a hospital for medical reasons, he should submit a letter from his doctor before the operation requesting prior approval.

Reversal of Vasectomy

Up to 5 percent of men who have vasectomies later decide they want to have a child. Reversal is a more complicated operation than vasectomy. It takes longer, costs more, and involves general anesthesia, a surgical team using microsurgery, and a hospital stay. To reverse a vasectomy, the surgeon attempts to reconnect each vas deferens in an extremely delicate operation. Channels only 1/100th of an inch in diameter must be rejoined.

The operation itself takes an hour or two. The surgeon makes an incision, examines the tubes, and tries to reconnect them with superfine sutures. The procedure requires a few days in the hospital and a few more at home for recuperation. The potential side effects and risks are similar to those associated with vasectomy.

HOW WELL DOES REVERSAL
OF VASECTOMY WORK?

Sometimes it is possible to reverse the operation, but there are no guarantees. Success in restoring fertility is uncertain. After vasectomy reversal, a man has a 16 to 79 percent chance of being able to cause pregnancy. Where a man's chances fall within this wide range depends on a number of factors, including:

Seven Common Questions Men Ask about Vasectomy

Will I be as masculine as I am now?

Yes. Vasectomy is not castration. Sterility is not impotence. The hormones that affect masculinity, beard, voice, sex drive, and other masculine traits are still made in testicles. They still flow throughout the body in the bloodstream.

Will vasectomy affect my sexual pleasure?

Erections, orgasms, and ejaculations will very likely be the same. Most men say they have greater sexual pleasure because they don't have to worry about causing an unwanted pregnancy. Many say there is no change.

How soon can I have sex again?

That depends on you. The general recommendation is to wait two to three days, and most men start again within a week. Others have sex sooner. Some wait longer. But remember, it takes about 15 to 20 ejaculations to clear sperm out of your system. Use another form of birth control for vaginal intercourse until a semen analysis shows that sperm are no longer in your seminal fluid.

Will there be "cum" when I "come"?

Yes. But there will be no sperm in the ejaculate. Your semen is between 2 and 5 percent sperm. The rest is seminal fluid from the prostate and other glands. The change in the amount of fluid is too little to notice.

- the length of time since the vasectomy was performed
- whether or not antisperm antibodies have developed
- the age of the woman partner with whom the man would like to have a child
- the method used for vasectomy
- the length and location of the segments of viable vas deferens that remain

Where do the sperm go after vasectomy?
They dissolve and are absorbed into the body. Dead and unused cells are absorbed by the body throughout life.

How much time will I have to take off work?
That depends on your general health, your attitude, and your job. Most men lose little or no time from work. A few need a day or two to rest. You will have to avoid strenuous labor or exercise for three to five days.

Rare complications may require more days at home; however, prompt medical attention should clear up any problems.

How much will it hurt?
You and your doctor will discuss which type of anesthetic to use. Local anesthetic is most usual. Sometimes a general anesthetic is called for. No pain is felt under general anesthesia because you are asleep. Some discomfort may be felt when the local anesthetic is injected or when the tubes are brought out of the scrotum through the incision. You may feel a dull ache in your groin or lower abdomen and a little queasiness or nausea.

As with any surgery, there's some discomfort after the operation. It will be different for each man, but most men say the pain is slight or moderate as opposed to excessive. An athletic supporter, ice bag, and Tylenol may help relieve the pain. There is less pain associated with no-scalpel procedures.

WHERE TO GET A REVERSAL OF VASECTOMY
AND WHAT IT COSTS

To inquire about a reversal, a man should contact the surgeon who performed the operation or another doctor. A local Planned Parenthood health center may also be able to provide a referral to a surgeon experienced in this procedure.

The average total cost of a reversal is about $10,000. The surgeon usually charges $1,600 to $5,000. Related costs include preliminary screening tests to see whether a man would be a good candidate for reversal and the fees for the operating room, the assistant surgeon, the anesthesiologist, and the hospital stay. Most health insurance plans will not pay for vasectomy reversals.

Tubal Sterilization—
Sterilization for Women

Tubal sterilization is permanent birth control for women. It is a surgical operation that is intended to cause sterility. More and more women today choose sterilization. They know that there is some chance of failure with any temporary method. They know that many temporary methods have side effects. And they know that most temporary methods can be inconvenient. Sterilization is often the answer for women who have completed their families and for women who do not want children. It is nearly 100 percent foolproof. And it does not decrease a woman's sexual pleasure.

About 600,000 tubal sterilizations are performed each year in the United States. More than half of them are performed shortly after childbirth or an abortion. Many women say they have enjoyed sex more after the operation because they are finally free of worry about unintended pregnancy. Their partners are often similarly relieved. In fact, women who have tubal sterilization have sexual intercourse more frequently after the operation than they did before the operation.

Tubal sterilization closes off the fallopian tubes, where eggs are fertilized by sperm. When the tubes are closed, sperm cannot reach the egg, and pregnancy cannot happen. The egg dissolves and is absorbed into the surrounding tissue.

Sterilization does not affect femininity. It is very unlikely that sterilization will affect a woman's sex organs or sexuality. No glands or organs will be removed or changed. All of the hormones will still be produced. The ovaries will release an egg every month. Menstrual cycles will most likely follow their usual patterns.

Mentally competent women can legally choose tubal sterilization in all 50 states. No one who is mentally competent can be forced to have the operation. Welfare benefits cannot be denied to women who refuse sterilization. Attempts to do so are against federal law.

Policies and practices about providing sterilization vary with individual doctors, hospitals, and health centers. The procedure may be difficult to arrange under some circumstances—for instance, if a woman is young, single, or childless.

Women do not need to have the consent of their husbands or other partners, but discussion with them is very important. Waiting periods are sometimes required to allow more time for thought before the operation. For federally funded tubal sterilizations, women must:

- be at least 21 years old
- observe a 30-day waiting period after signing a statement of informed consent
- be free of the influence of alcohol or other drugs at the time of consent
- reapply if the procedure is postponed for more than 180 days

How Well Tubal Sterilization Works

Tubal sterilization is one of the most effective methods of birth control for sexually active women—only Norplant is as effective. A woman and her partner will need no other contraceptive after a successful tubal sterilization.

A woman must consider the operation permanent. While it is

possible to reverse sterilization in some cases, the decision not to have a child in the future must be firm. So a woman must be absolutely sure she will never change her mind or regret her choice—no matter how her life changes.

Tubal sterilization works immediately and is more than 99 percent effective. In very rare cases, tubes may reconnect by themselves, and pregnancy may occur. Such rare pregnancies may be ectopic—develop outside the uterus (womb)—and require emergency surgery. Of 1,000 women who have tubal sterilizations, no more than 5 will become pregnant in the first year. About 1 woman of every 1,000 will become pregnant each year for the next 10 years or so. About 50 percent of those pregnancies will be ectopic.

Tubal sterilization offers no protection against sexually transmitted infections.

Sterilization will not cause symptoms of menopause (change of life) or make menopause happen earlier.

In about 1 out of every 100 attempted tubal sterilization procedures, it is found to be impossible to block the fallopian tubes. The tubes may have been badly scarred from disease or there may be some other condition that makes it impossible for the surgeon to complete the operation.

Women Who May Want to Consider Sterilization

Women may consider sterilization for many reasons, including the following:

- They want to enjoy having sex without causing pregnancy.
- They don't want to have a child in the future.
- They and their partners agree that their family is complete and no more children are wanted.
- They and their partners have concerns about the side effects of other methods.
- Other methods are unacceptable to them.
- Their health would be threatened by a future pregnancy.
- They don't want to pass on a hereditary illness or disability.

Women Who Should Not Consider Sterilization

Sterilization should not be considered by women under the following conditions:

- They are in their teens or early 20s.
- They may want to have a child in the future.
- They are being pressured by a partner, friends, or family. *The woman* must want the operation.
- They want to resolve a temporary problem. Marital or sexual problems, short-term mental or physical illnesses, financial worries, being out of work, and other circumstances that may change are not good reasons for tubal sterilization.
- They have not considered possible changes in their lives, such as divorce, remarriage, or death of children.
- They have not discussed tubal sterilization fully with their partners.
- They are under too much stress to make such an important lifelong decision.
- They are concerned that a tubal sterilization may affect their femininity or their sexual pleasure.
- They are counting on reversal if they change their minds.

Alternatives to Tubal Sterilization

A woman should consider all other methods before she chooses sterilization. The Pill, Norplant, Depo-Provera, and IUDs are more than 95 percent effective. Most women can use one of them with little risk of serious complications. Other methods that have little or no side effects are diaphragms, cervical caps, condoms, vaginal foams, jellies, suppositories, periodic abstinence, and fertility awareness methods. But all these are less reliable than sterilization.

A woman's partner may want to consider sterilization. Sterilization for men is called vasectomy. Vasectomy is simpler, costs less, and has fewer risks than tubal sterilization. But vasectomy also must be considered permanent. Both partners should think carefully about what sterilization will mean for both of them before they make their decision.

Methods for Tubal Sterilization

Tubal sterilizations are performed in hospitals or in clinics with surgical units. They are done under local or general anesthesia. Closing the tubes for sterilization can be done in several ways. Sometimes the tubes are closed off by tying and cutting (tubal ligation), sealing (cautery or electrocoagulation), or applying clips, clamps, or rings. Sometimes a small piece of each tube is removed.

A woman's health condition may indicate which procedure is better suited for her. Previous surgery and body weight are two important factors to consider. Women who have had certain types of abdominal surgery may not be able to have tubal sterilization. A woman should consult her health care provider if she has any questions.

Some Factors to Consider

Hospitalization may be appropriate for a woman who wants tubal sterilization if she:

- weighs more than 50 percent over her ideal body weight
- has had a serious infection of the abdominal cavity—peritonitis—especially after a ruptured appendix
- has had pelvic inflammatory disease (PID) in the previous year
- has had three or more episodes of PID at any time in the past
- has had more than one laparotomy, major abdominal surgery, for any reason, including surgery of the fallopian tubes or cesarean section

Sterilization may be postponed for a woman who:

- may need to have a laparoscopy, minor abdominal surgery in which a small scope and other instruments are inserted into the abdomen to diagnose or treat certain conditions; a hysterectomy, the removal of the uterus; or a laparotomy for endometriosis in the near future
- has had one or more large fibroids

Getting a Tubal Sterilization

FIRST STEP—THE MEDICAL EXAM

Before deciding whether a woman is a good candidate for a tubal sterilization, the doctor will discuss her medical history with her. She will have a physical examination, including a breast exam and pelvic exam. Samples of blood and urine will be taken for laboratory tests. Unless she's had a normal Pap test within the past nine months, a Pap test will also be necessary. The woman will be tested for sexually transmitted infections and for pregnancy. Many practitioners recommend a pregnancy test within 48 hours of the procedure.

- is being monitored or treated for a cystic mass in an ovary
- has an abnormal result on her Pap test

Other health conditions that may affect whether or not a woman is a good candidate for outpatient tubal sterilization include:
- asthma
- diabetes
- heart disease
- high blood pressure
- hepatitis
- chronic kidney (renal) disease
- systemic lupus erythematosus (an autoimmune disease)
- any condition that requires taking anticoagulant medication, which thins the blood and could make surgery dangerous and recovery more difficult

These conditions may require extra medical precautions or special anesthetic care.

It may be a good idea for a woman to ask her partner to have a semen analysis before planning a tubal sterilization. Many men are sterile without knowing it. If a man has had mumps during adulthood or if he has any other reason to think he may be sterile, the possibility should be discussed with the doctor. If a woman's partner is sterile, tubal sterilization may not be necessary for her at that time, if ever.

A woman's doctor will consider her psychological as well as her physical health to determine if she is a good candidate for tubal sterilization. Often the first step is counseling by the surgeon or someone else who is knowledgeable about the subject, such as a nurse or social worker.

The counselor will make sure the woman understands what a tubal sterilization involves and that she has considered her other contraceptive options. She may be asked to consider how she would feel if, after her tubal sterilization, she lost her current partner and took another who wanted a child. What if her existing child or children died?

Talking with other women who have had tubal sterilizations may be helpful. If a woman doesn't have a friend or relative she can ask, the doctor may provide her with the name of someone who may be of help.

Once she has decided to proceed, a woman will be asked to sign consent forms attesting that she understands all aspects of what will and may happen before, during, and after a tubal sterilization.

SECOND STEP—PERSONAL PREPARATIONS

Before a tubal sterilization, a woman should:

- Arrange for someone to drive her home after surgery.
- Arrange to take some time off work after the operation. A woman should talk with her surgeon about her recovery and how long she can expect to be out of work. The time needed will depend on the procedure decided upon. She should expect to need at least a couple of days off her feet at home.
- Arrange for someone to be with the children. She should be sure

that someone is around to give a hand for at least the first 24 hours after returning home. Even if the children are away, a woman may want an adult around to make things more comfortable.

- Fill any prescription for painkillers her doctor thinks she may need. A woman should be sure she has the medication before the surgery. She will not want to pick it up afterward.

- Ask the doctor for a telephone number that can be called 24 hours a day after the surgery in case of an emergency.

- Avoid aspirin or any medications containing aspirin during the week before surgery. Aspirin thins the blood and interferes with clotting. If a woman ordinarily takes aspirin or any other blood thinner, such as warfarin (Coumadin), for a medical condition, she should consult her doctor.

- Ask to have a trained counselor at her side during the operation if she is going to have local anesthesia and will be awake during the surgery. A woman should be sure to request a counselor before the day of the procedure.

- Avoid drinking alcohol or taking any other drugs during the day before surgery, unless her doctor has approved doing so. A woman may get permission to take a mild sedative on the day of the procedure to stay calm. This may help relieve stress that can tighten the muscles and increase pain.

- Avoid eating or drinking anything except a little water for at least eight hours before surgery.

- Contact the physician if a cold, fever, flu symptoms, or any other infection develops—especially a reproductive tract infection—shortly before the appointment. She may have to reschedule.

- Cancel the surgery if she has any last-minute doubts. A woman should not go through with it just because the arrangements have been made. She should cancel the arrangements and think them over.

- Wash with extra care on the morning of the surgery, possibly with an antibacterial soap such as pHisoHex® or Betadine®. Wash the vulva, pubic hair, and navel thoroughly.

Just before going into the operating room, a woman will be asked to urinate. Some surgical teams insert a catheter into the urethra to drain urine from the bladder during surgery. Because catheterization increases the chance of infection, a woman may want to tell her surgeon beforehand that she prefers that a catheter not be used.

If local anesthesia is being used for the procedure, a woman may be injected with a tranquilizer an hour before the surgery. Or she may be given a mild sedative 30 to 60 minutes before the procedure. Pubic hair may be shaved at this time. Local anesthetics will be injected around the navel and into the tissues under it. The woman will feel only the first of the injections.

If general anesthesia is being used for the procedure, the medication will be delivered into a vein in the arm through an intravenous tube. When a woman is unconscious, the anesthesiologist will insert a tube through her mouth into the windpipe to help her breathe. This procedure may result in a sore throat for a couple of days after surgery.

A woman's heart and lungs will be monitored with various equipment throughout the surgery.

THIRD STEP—THE PROCEDURE

There are a number of different procedures used for tubal sterilization. The most common involve an incision made through the abdomen. Less commonly, the incision is made in the vagina.

Abdominal Procedures for Tubal Sterilization

- **Laparoscopy.** Laparoscopy is often performed in outpatient surgical clinics. It takes 20 to 30 minutes. Very little scarring occurs, and women often go home the same day. A few days of rest at home should be sufficient for a full recovery. They may have sexual intercourse as soon as they feel comfortable about it.

  In this procedure, the surgeon makes a tiny incision under the navel. The surgeon inserts a laparoscope through the incision. The laparoscope is a long, thin, hollow, flexible instrument with a tiny camera at the far end and a lens for the surgeon to look through. The surgeon also watches the procedure on a screen in the operating room.

Other instruments can be inserted through the laparoscope or through a second tiny incision made in the lower abdomen. One of the instruments is a tube through which a harmless gas (carbon dioxide or nitrous oxide) is pumped into the abdomen, inflating it to give the surgeon a better view and more room to work.

The surgeon locates the fallopian tubes, cuts them, and closes them off. The gas is slowly released from the abdomen through the laparoscope. The laparoscope is removed. The doctor gently but firmly presses down on the abdomen to expel as much gas as possible.

The incision is closed with a few small stitches. The doctor may use self-absorbing sutures that dissolve in about a week or nonabsorbable sutures that will be removed five to seven days later.

The incision is small enough to be covered with one or two Band-Aids®. That's why a laparoscopy is sometimes called Band-Aid surgery. It's also called belly button surgery because the incision is often made near the navel.

- **Mini-laparotomy.** Mini-laparotomy ("mini-lap") is another common method of sterilization. A local anesthetic is often used, and the operation can take place in a doctor's office or clinic. Mini-laparotomy is often performed after childbirth. Mini-laparotomy is more invasive than laparoscopy. No gas or visualizing instrument is used in mini-laparotomy. Women usually recover in a few days. Doctors will advise when sexual intercourse can be resumed.

   In this procedure, a small incision is made just above the pubic hair. If the operation takes place within 48 hours after childbirth, the incision is made just below the navel. Using special tools, the surgeon eases the fallopian tubes through the incision one at a time, then cuts and closes them off. The mini-lap can be done in connection with childbirth, when the uterus and fallopian tubes are higher in the abdomen than usual and are easier for the surgeon to reach. A mini-lap can also be done immediately after an abortion.

Pain may be more intense or last longer than after a laparoscopy. Recovery takes a few days. Mini-laparotomy is not appropriate for women who are very overweight.

- **Laparotomy.** Laparotomy is major surgery, less commonly used than mini-laparotomy and laparoscopy. Laparotomy was the most commonly used method before new technology made laparoscopies and mini-laparotomies possible. The operation requires general or spinal anesthesia. A woman may need to be hospitalized for five to seven days and may take several weeks at home to completely recover. If the procedure is done after delivery, the woman's hospital stay may be extended by one or two days. The rate of recovery affects when sexual intercourse can be resumed.

  In this procedure, the surgeon makes a two-to-five-inch incision in the abdomen just above the pubic hair, then locates and closes off the tubes. Because the incision is larger than the incisions for laparoscopy and mini-laparotomy, more stitches are needed to close it.

  Pain during the first 24 to 48 hours is relieved with medication. Laparotomies may be appropriate for women whose tubes are scarred from endometriosis, pelvic inflammatory disease, or previous surgery because laparotomy allows closer examination of the tubes. Sterilization can sometimes be done when an abdominal incision is made to correct other conditions.

Vaginal Procedures for Tubal Sterilization

Vaginal procedures are not performed very frequently in the United States. Fewer and fewer surgeons are trained in the procedures.

- **Culdoscopy.** The surgeon makes an incision in the vagina. Then the surgeon inserts a culdoscope (an instrument with a light on the end) through the incision. The tubes are located, brought into view, closed off, and returned to their normal positions.

- **Colpotomy.** The surgeon makes an incision in the vagina. No visualizing instrument is used. The tubes are located, brought into view, closed off, and returned to their normal positions.

Culdoscopy and colpotomy have become much less popular in the United States and Europe since the advent of laparoscopy, although they are still widely used in some countries. These procedures take 15 to 30 minutes, and women usually go home the same day. It may take a few days at home for them to recuperate. Sexual intercourse is usually postponed until the incision is completely healed, as advised by the doctor. This may take several weeks.

There are no visible scars with these procedures. However, there may be more risk of serious infection than with other procedures because the incision in the vagina can bring up bacteria from the vaginal area. Also, the failure rate (about 2 percent) is higher than for abdominal procedures. Some women experience painful intercourse after being sterilized through the vagina.

Blocking the Ends of the Tubes

There are several techniques doctors use to close the ends of the tubes to prevent them from reconnecting, which is called recanalization. Recanalization is rare but accounts for a significant proportion of failures associated with tubal sterilization.

- **Tying (ligation).** Once the ends have been cut, the doctor folds them back and ties off each one with surgical thread. Ligation can be used with laparotomy, but not with vaginal procedures, laparoscopy, or mini-lap. This method was used for so long that "tubal ligation" and "having your tubes tied" have become synonymous with sterilization for women.
- **Metal clips and silastic rings.** The cut ends are closed off with clips or rings. Damage to the tubes caused by clips and rings reduces the risk of recanalization and the chances of reversal. Pressure on the tubes from these methods can cause painful cramps for several hours after the surgery.
- **Electrocoagulation.** Special forceps are used to administer a high-frequency electric current that quickly coagulates the inner tissue of the tube, sealing the end with a scar.

FOURTH STEP—RECUPERATING

A woman will rest in a supervised recovery room for at least two hours after surgery that involves a local anesthetic. She should be able to walk without assistance, be alert enough to understand instructions about taking care of herself (these may also be provided in writing), and be able to urinate without a catheter before she's allowed to leave. Someone will have to be available to drive her home. Before she leaves for home, she should be sure she has a 24-hour telephone number for emergency calls.

If a woman has had general anesthesia, she should remain in the hospital for at least five hours or overnight. She will probably feel nauseated for a day or so. She may take one or two nonaspirin pain relievers every four to six hours or whatever medications her doctor recommends or prescribes.

The discomfort felt after the operation depends on general health, the type of surgery performed, and the woman's tolerance for pain. She is less likely to feel dizzy, nauseated, bloated, gassy, or sore in the shoulder, or to have abdominal cramping with local anesthesia than with general anesthesia. A headache often follows spinal anesthesia but not an epidural.

A woman should take it very easy for at least 24 hours and fairly easy for a week. Even if she feels terrific, she should not do any heavy lifting for at least a week after surgery. This may be difficult at times, but it's important for a smooth recovery. She should allow her family and friends to give her a hand.

The doctor will probably allow a woman to shower about 48 hours after surgery. She should be sure to pat her incision dry after bathing.

A woman will probably be asked to return to the doctor's office or clinic a week after surgery to make sure she is healing well. If the surgeon has used nonabsorbable sutures, they will be removed at that time.

FIFTH STEP—RESUMING NORMAL ACTIVITIES

With her doctor's permission, a woman should probably be able to return to her usual schedule, including work or sports, within a week after surgery. If she has had an abdominal procedure, she will be able to resume sexual intercourse after a couple of days or whenever she feels up to it—most women wait a week or more. A woman who has a vaginal procedure or sterilization after childbirth will have to wait longer—up to several weeks.

Risks Associated with Tubal Sterilization

Tubal sterilization is low-risk surgery. Complications can occur with any kind of surgery. The complications that can occur during or after sterilization are:

- bleeding
- infection
- reaction to the anesthetic

Infection is rare, but it occurs more frequently after sterilization performed through the vagina. Infections are treated with antibiotics. Very rarely, the bowel, blood vessels, bladder, or uterus are injured. Major surgery may be required to repair this.

Complications may develop in 1 to 4 percent of sterilizations performed through the abdomen. They may develop in 2 to 13 percent of sterilizations performed through the vagina. Deaths resulting from tubal sterilization are extremely rare—the rate is about 4 per 100,000.

If gas is used in the procedure, it will take two to seven days to completely leave the system. Meanwhile, women may experience some pain or discomfort in the chest, shoulders, or pelvic area.

Regret is rare after tubal sterilization. Women who are sterilized are no different psychologically from women who are not sterilized.

A woman should contact her doctor immediately if she:

- develops a fever
- has pus or bleeding from an incision
- has severe, continuous abdominal pain
- has fainting spells

Pregnancy and Tubal Sterilization

About half of the pregnancies that occur after sterilization are ectopic—they develop outside the uterus. Ectopic pregnancies must be removed or they will cause fatal complications.

SIGNS OF PREGNANCY:

- missed period or unusually light period
- nausea and vomiting
- breast tenderness
- fatigue

SIGNS OF ECTOPIC PREGNANCY:

- severe pain on one or both sides of the lower abdomen
- abdominal pain and spotting, especially after a missed menstrual period or a very light one
- faint or dizzy feeling

If a woman thinks she may have an ectopic pregnancy and can't reach her doctor, she should go to a hospital emergency room quickly.

Higher-Risk Surgery—Hysterectomy

Hysterectomy is the removal of the uterus. It is major surgery and is not usually used for sterilization. It is used to correct serious medical conditions. Hysterectomy ends menstruation as well the possibility of pregnancy. It does not necessarily affect the fallopian tubes. However, some medical conditions also call for the removal of a tube and/or ovary, on one side or both.

Hysterectomy is performed through the abdomen or vagina, and sometimes a combined approach is used. Following hysterectomy, a woman needs to spend several days in the hospital and usually several weeks at home recuperating. She should abstain from sexual intercourse from four to six weeks, until the doctor advises it is all right.

Complications after hysterectomy occur in 10 to 20 percent of cases. Because hysterectomy is usually performed on women who have a significant medical condition, the risk of death is much greater than it is for tubal sterilization—300 to 500 per 100,000 cases. The cost is also considerably greater.

Where to Get Tubal Sterilization and What It Costs

A tubal sterilization may be arranged through a family health care provider, health maintenance organization, local hospital, local public health department, or local Planned Parenthood health center. An appointment with the nearest Planned Parenthood health center may be scheduled by calling toll-free, 800-230-PLAN.

Information about tubal sterilization is also available from AVSC (Access to Voluntary and Safe Contraception International), 79 Madison Ave., 7th Floor, New York, NY 10016; 212-561-8000, or the American College of Obstetricians and Gynecologists, 409 12th St., SW, Washington, DC 20024; 202-638-5577.

(continued on page 208)

Advantages of Tubal Sterilization

- Tubal sterilization provides permanent, highly effective contraception.
- Tubal sterilization is inexpensive in the long term.
- Tubal sterilization is a relatively simple surgery that can usually be done under local anesthesia.
- Tubal sterilization has no proven, significant, long-term, medical side effects.
- Tubal sterilization offers great privacy.
- Tubal sterilization does not rely on partner compliance.
- Tubal sterilization does not interrupt sexual activity.

Disadvantages of Tubal Sterilization

- Tubal sterilization is a surgical procedure.
- Women who choose tubal sterilization will experience short-term pain and discomfort.
- Reversal is expensive and cannot be guaranteed.
- Tubal sterilization offers no protection against sexually transmitted infections.
- Tubal sterilization is expensive in the short term.

Common Questions Women Ask about Tubal Sterilization

Will sterilization end an existing pregnancy?
No. Sterilization will not be performed if you are pregnant.

Will sterilization cause menopause?
No. Sterilization does not cause menopause or any of its symptoms.

Will sterilization prevent menopause?
No. You will still experience menopause later in life.

Will I still have a period?
Yes. Your menstrual cycle and flow should be the same after the operation as they were before. However, if you were using birth control pills or Depo-Provera before the surgery, it may take a while for your cycle to get back to normal.

What happens to the eggs?
An egg is released each month. It dissolves and is absorbed by the body. Other dead and unused cells are absorbed naturally by the body throughout life.

Will I be as feminine?
Yes. The hormones that affect hair, voice, sex drive, muscle tone, breast size, and other feminine characteristics are still made in your ovaries. They will still flow throughout the body in the bloodstream.

Will I gain weight or develop facial hair?
No. Sterilization does not cause weight gain or facial hair.

Will sterilization hurt?
A general or local anesthetic will be used. The choice depends on your physical condition and the method of sterilization being used. Local anesthesia is much safer than general anesthesia because there is less risk of serious complications, including death.

General anesthesia is entirely painless, and you will not remain conscious. When a local anesthetic is injected, you may feel some pressure. The pain is relieved with medications and sedatives. You will remain conscious but sleepy. You will feel little or no discomfort during the procedure.

How soon can I have sexual intercourse again?

Ask your doctor's advice. Do not have intercourse until you feel comfortable about it. It usually takes about a week after abdominal sterilization. You will have to wait at least four weeks after a vaginal sterilization or sterilization after childbirth.

Will sterilization decrease my sexual pleasure?

No. In fact, many women and men report that they have less tension about unwanted pregnancy after sterilization. They feel that the lack of tension increases their sexual pleasure.

Can sterilization be reversed?

If you are thinking about reversal, don't have a tubal sterilization. Reversal procedures require complicated surgery and cost thousands of dollars. Even though tubes can sometimes be rejoined, pregnancy cannot be guaranteed. Many women cannot even attempt reversals because there is not enough of their tubes left in the reproductive tract.

How soon can I go back to work?

That depends on your general health, your attitude, your job, and the method of sterilization that you had. With the most common methods—mini-laparotomy and laparoscopy—recovery is usually complete in a day or two. You may want to take it easy for the next week or so. In any case, you should avoid heavy lifting for about one week.

For the most common procedures, the cost is about $1,000 to $2,500. Some clinics and doctors adjust fees on a sliding scale according to income. Procedures that require hospitalization are more expensive.

Blue Cross and Blue Shield and some private health insurance policies pay some or most of the cost. In about 35 states, Medicaid pays but puts some restrictions on patient eligibility. A 30-day waiting period is required from the signing of the consent form to the time that federally funded operations are performed. Federally funded sterilizations may not be performed on anyone under 21 or anyone incapable of legal consent. A woman should check with her local welfare department to see if she is covered.

The cost of hysterectomy is considerably higher. Medicaid and federal funds (such as for federal employees, including members of the armed forces and their families) won't pay for a hysterectomy that's being performed only for sterilization.

Reversal of Tubal Sterilization

About 1 out of 1,000 women who have been sterilized ask to have the operation reversed so that they can have a child. Reversal is more difficult and complicated than sterilization. It takes longer, costs more, and involves general anesthesia, a surgical team using microsurgery, a one-week hospital stay, and two to three weeks of recovery time at home.

To explore whether reversal is the right step for a woman to take, a surgeon will review her medical history, including the medical files from her sterilization. She will have a physical examination, followed by blood and urine tests done in a laboratory. The woman's partner will also be examined to be sure that he is fertile.

HOW WELL REVERSAL OF TUBAL STERILIZATION WORKS

Sometimes it is possible to reverse the operation, but there are no guarantees. Success in restoring fertility is uncertain. After reversal of a tubal sterilization, a woman has a 43 to 88 percent chance of being able to become pregnant. Where a woman's chances fall within this range depends on a number of factors, including:

- the way the tubes were closed during the sterilization procedure
- how much undamaged tube remains to be reconnected
- the health and age of the woman
- the health and fertility of the partner with whom she intends to have a child

WHERE TO GET A TUBAL STERILIZATION REVERSED AND WHAT IT COSTS

A woman should contact the surgeon who performed the operation to inquire about a reversal. A major hospital, gynecologist, or local Planned Parenthood center may also be able to refer a woman to a surgeon experienced in this procedure.

The average total cost of a reversal is about $10,000. The surgeon's fees are usually about $5,000. Related costs include preliminary screening tests to see whether a woman would be a good candidate for reversal and the fees for the operating room, the assistant surgeon, the anesthesiologist, and the hospital stay. Not all health insurance plans pay for sterilization reversals.

10

◆

When Contraception Fails—Pregnancy Options

- *"What If I'm Pregnant?"*
- *What about Raising a Child?*
- *What about Placing the Baby for Adoption?*
- *What about Abortion?*

Half of the 3.3 million unintended pregnancies that occur in the United States every year are due to contraceptive failure—either the method fails or, more likely, it is used inconsistently or incorrectly. (Women who do not use contraception are nearly six times more likely to have an unintended pregnancy than women who do use contraception.) Most American women want to become mothers when they are ready and can plan for it, but young or middle-aged, women often face difficult decisions when pregnancy is unplanned—whether or not it is due to contraceptive failure.

"What If I'm Pregnant?"

A woman may ask herself this question at many times in her life—especially when her period is late. If you think you are pregnant, you may be asking yourself lots of other questions, too.

- "Is having a baby the best choice for me?"
- "Is adding another child the best for our family?"
- "Is raising a child by myself the best choice for me?"
- "Is raising a child with a partner the best choice for me?"
- "Is placing the baby for adoption the best choice for me?"
- "Is having an abortion the best choice for me?"

If you think you are pregnant, you will want to choose what's right for you, but first, be sure you are pregnant. A urine or blood test performed by a clinician is the surest way to find out. You can get home pregnancy tests at most drugstores and wherever feminine hygiene products are sold. They are simple to use, but they may be inaccurate—especially if not used properly.

If you use a home pregnancy test, be sure to read the directions carefully before using it, then be sure to follow them exactly. To be sure about whether you are pregnant, have your pregnancy test done at your health care provider's office, a Planned Parenthood health center, or another family planning clinic. For an appointment with the Planned Parenthood health center nearest you, call 800-230-PLAN.

If your test indicates that you are pregnant, you will also need a physical exam to be absolutely sure. The exam will also tell how long you have been pregnant. Then you will need to decide what you want to do.

If you are pregnant, you have to consider your options. There is no right or wrong choice for everyone. Only you can decide which choice is right for you. Some women know immediately what they will do if they have an unintended pregnancy. Many need to consider their options over time. Here are the options:

- You can choose to have a baby and raise the child.

- You can choose to have a baby and place the child for adoption.
- You can choose to end the pregnancy.

If you are considering pregnancy options for an unintended pregnancy, here are some questions you might ask yourself to help you make your decision. Consider each of your choices carefully. Take your time and ask yourself:

- Which choice(s) could I live with?
- Which choice(s) would be impossible for me?
- How would each choice affect my everyday life?
- What would each choice mean to the people closest to me?
- What is going on in my life that affects my choice?
- How will another child affect our family?
- What are my plans for the future?
- What are my spiritual and moral beliefs?
- What do I believe is best for me in the long run?
- What will be best for our family?
- What can I afford?

Talk about your feelings with your partner, someone in your family, or a trusted friend. All family planning clinics have specially trained counselors. These counselors can talk with you about your options. Your counselor will try to make sure that you are not being pressured into any decision against your will. You may bring your husband, partner, parents, or someone else, if you wish.

To make the choice that will suit you best, find out as much as you can about all your choices.

"How Soon Do I Have to Decide What to Do?"

If there is a chance that you will continue the pregnancy, you should begin prenatal care as soon as possible. You should have a medical exam early in your pregnancy to make sure that you are healthy and that the pregnancy is normal.

If you are considering abortion, you should make your decision as

How to Find the Right Health Center

Be sure to look for a health center that will give you complete information about your options. If you need help finding one, call Planned Parenthood at 800-230-PLAN for a referral. Beware that "crisis pregnancy centers" are anti-abortion propaganda centers. They are very likely to try to influence your decision.

- They may perform your pregnancy tests without medical supervision.
- They won't give you complete and correct information about all options.
- They will try to frighten you with films that are designed to keep you from choosing abortion.
- They will lie to you about the medical and emotional effects of abortion.
- They may tell you that you are not pregnant, even if you are, to fool you into continuing your pregnancy without knowing. The delay would make abortion more risky and keep you from getting prenatal care.
- They will discourage you from using the most reliable methods of birth control.

soon as possible. Abortion is very safe, but the risks increase the longer a pregnancy goes on. Surgical abortion is usually performed between the sixth and eighth weeks of pregnancy. Medical abortion may be performed much earlier—as soon as a pregnancy is confirmed.

While you are deciding what to do, take good care of yourself. If you do decide to have a child, you will want it to be healthy and well. Good prenatal care is very important for a baby's health.

- Get enough good food—fruits, vegetables, cereals, breads, beans, rice, and dairy products as well as fish, meat, and poultry.
- Keep your body in good shape. Stay active and get regular exercise.

- Get plenty of sleep.
- Do not smoke.
- Do not drink alcohol or drinks with caffeine, such as coffee and cola.
- Do not eat junk food.
- Do not take any drugs or medications—even aspirin—without checking with your health care provider.
- Drink eight glasses of water every day.

You can get complete information about prenatal care and how to pay for it from your family doctor, your local Planned Parenthood health center, other family planning clinics, women's health centers, and your state's department of family services.

What about Raising a Child?

One of your choices is to continue your pregnancy and raise a child. Being a parent is exciting, rewarding, and demanding. It can help you grow, understand yourself better, and enhance your life.

You have choices, though, in how you raise a child. You may want to raise a child with a partner. Or you may want to raise a child without a partner.

Parenting with a Partner

Most of us look forward to finding a life partner—someone with whom we can share the pleasures, responsibilities, and difficulties of family life. If you are in a committed relationship like marriage and have already established a family, you may find warm and loving support from your partner and children as you consider expanding the family.

If you are going to establish a family with your partner, you may want to consider marriage. Marriage is a serious legal contract binding both partners. Each one accepts legal as well as moral and emo-

Here are some things to consider if you are thinking about parenting with a partner:

True False

[ ]   [ ]   1. I'll get what I want in life if I start a family now.

[ ]   [ ]   2. My/his parents are pushing us into marriage.

[ ]   [ ]   3. Having a child will strengthen our family.

[ ]   [ ]   4. We're both financially and emotionally ready for a child.

[ ]   [ ]   5. We get upset when we talk about a long-term, committed relationship.

[ ]   [ ]   6. I know what to expect of my partner, and he knows what to expect of me.

[ ]   [ ]   7. Marriage will help me feel less guilty about having sex.

[ ]   [ ]   8. He's agreed to help out with child care and housework, too.

[ ]   [ ]   9. We'd stay together even if I weren't pregnant.

[ ]   [ ]   10. I'm prepared to be a single parent if things don't work out between us.

Think about what your answers mean to you. You may want to discuss your thinking with your partner, someone else in your family, a trusted friend, or your counselor.

tional obligations to the other. Every state has its own laws about marriage. If you are under 18, contact your local marriage license bureau or consult your religious adviser to find out about the laws in your state.

Consider premarital counseling if marriage is one of your choices. Taking the time to talk about marriage with a counselor can make a big difference, no matter how old you and your partner may be. See a private counselor or get counseling through your church, temple, mosque, or some other community service. Family counseling is also beneficial for all couples, married or not, whenever they consider beginning or expanding a family.

With or without marriage, a life partnership can succeed if both people:

- are deeply committed to make it work
- understand what each expects from the relationship

Having a child can bring joy, stability, and many other rewards to a relationship. A child can also strain the best relationship. If your commitment is not solid, the relationship may fail.

Parenting without a Partner

The challenge of raising a child alone can also be exciting and rewarding. It is easier if you find and use all the support you can. Before you decide to become a *single* parent, be sure to let family and friends know that you hope for their support.

Even with the help of your family and friends, being a single parent is not easy. It is time-consuming and often complicated and frustrating. Your child's needs will constantly change, and so will your ability to meet those needs. To help you through these changes, you may want to consider counseling, which you may find out about from your local department of children's services.

Your child will look to you for love and care—all day, every day. And you can take great pleasure helping your child grow into a happy, independent, and responsible adult. But there will be no breaks. If the child is ill or disabled, even greater effort may be required. It takes years for children to become responsible for themselves. And convenient, affordable child care is difficult to find.

It takes a lot of money to raise a child. Earning a living for yourself and your child will be a real challenge—even if you have finished school and have a good job. Your own parent(s) may find it hard to help you out with all the bills. Welfare payments barely cover the basics.

Because your child will need you so much, you may become

Here are some things to consider if you are thinking about parenting without a partner:

True False

[ ] [ ] 1. Loving my baby will get me through hard times.

[ ] [ ] 2. I'm being pressured to keep the baby.

[ ] [ ] 3. I'm willing to put school and career on hold.

[ ] [ ] 4. I'll be more dependent on other people.

[ ] [ ] 5. Money won't be a problem.

[ ] [ ] 6. My baby will give me all the love I need.

[ ] [ ] 7. I know someone who is always available and who I can trust to take care of the child when I'm at work or school or when I'm ill.

[ ] [ ] 8. Having another child will strengthen my family.

[ ] [ ] 9. I'll find a life partner more easily with a child.

[ ] [ ] 10. My family and friends will be supportive.

Think about what your answers mean to you. You may want to discuss your thinking with someone else in your family, a trusted friend, or your counselor.

more dependent on your own family and friends—for help with the child, for money, and for emotional support. You may have to give up a lot of freedom to be a good single parent. On the other hand, because you will not have to make compromises with a partner, you can raise the child as you wish—with your values, principles, and beliefs.

Parenting requires lots of love and unlimited energy and patience. There will be times when you may feel that you are not doing a good job at it. To feel good about being a single parent, it must be what you want to do—for a long time. If you have other children, you already know what that means. If you don't, talk with a single mother or with a counselor who works with single mothers.

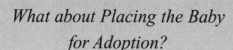

What about Placing the Baby for Adoption?

One of your choices is to complete your pregnancy and let someone else raise your child. Many women who make this choice are happy knowing that their children are loved and living in good homes. But some women find that the pain of being separated from their children is deeper and more long-lasting than they expected. Women who relinquish their children for adoption seem to have more regret than women who chose other options.

There are two kinds of adoption:

- **Closed Adoption.** In this, the names of the birth mother and the adoptive parents are kept secret from one another.
- **Open Adoption.** In this, the names of the birth mother and the adoptive parents are known to one another. The birth mother may select the adoptive parents for her child. She and the adoptive parents may choose to get to know one another. They may also choose to have an ongoing relationship.

Adoption is legal and binding whether it is open or closed. Few adoptions are reversed by the courts. You will have to sign relinquishment papers some time after your baby is born. In most states, minors do not need a parent's consent to choose adoption. However, the child's father can demand custody of the child unless he signs release papers before the adoption takes place. Adoption laws are different in every state. Find out in advance what they are in your state. Talk with an adoption counselor or lawyer before deciding on any arrangement. Be sure to read everything *very* carefully before you sign. It is always best to have a lawyer review all documents first. All adoptions must be approved by a judge in a family or surrogate court.

Adoption is arranged in three ways:

- **Agency (Licensed) Adoption.** The birth parents relinquish their child to the agency. The agency places the child into the adoptive home.
- **Independent (Unlicensed) Adoption.** The birth parents relinquish their child directly into the adoptive home.
- **Adoption by Relatives.** The court grants legal adoption to relatives.

Thousands of women and men are waiting to adopt newborn children. However, there is no guarantee that homes will be found for all children waiting to be adopted. This is especially true of children of color and children who are disabled.

Agency (Licensed) Adoption

You can place your child through a public or private agency that is licensed by the government. These agencies:

- provide counseling
- handle legal matters
- make hospital arrangements for your child's birth
- select a home for your child
- refer you to agencies that may help you financially

Sometimes an agency is able to help find a home for you during your pregnancy. In agency adoption, your name and the adoptive parents' names are usually kept secret. However, some licensed agencies also offer various open adoption options.

Most religious organizations can help you locate a licensed adoption agency. You can also look in the Yellow Pages under "adoption agencies" and "social service organizations." Or you can contact your state, county, or local department of family or child services, or your local Planned Parenthood center.

The National Committee for Adoption hotline can refer you to licensed agencies in your area. Call 202-328-8072. If you are pregnant, you can call collect. Or you can write to the National Committee for Adoption, 1940 17th St., NW, Washington, DC 20009.

Independent (Unlicensed) Adoption

You can arrange an independent adoption through a doctor or lawyer or someone else who knows a couple that wants to adopt. Some states have private, independent adoption centers that provide counseling. These centers are run by women and men who want to adopt. Independent adoptions are not legal in some states because there is a risk that birth mothers and adoptive parents may be exploited.

An independent adoption is usually an open adoption. The adoptive parents will often agree to pay your hospital and medical bills until the child is born. They may even pay your living expenses during that time. Usually the adoptive parents hire one lawyer to repre-

---

Here are some things to consider if you are thinking about adoption:

True False

[ ] [ ] 1. I can accept my child living with someone else.

[ ] [ ] 2. Going through pregnancy and delivery won't change my mind.

[ ] [ ] 3. I'm willing to have good prenatal care.

[ ] [ ] 4. I'm choosing adoption because abortion scares me.

[ ] [ ] 5. The child's birth father will approve of adoption.

[ ] [ ] 6. No one is pressuring me to choose adoption.

[ ] [ ] 7. I'll know my child is being treated well.

[ ] [ ] 8. I won't be jealous of the adoptive parents.

[ ] [ ] 9. I care what other people will think.

[ ] [ ] 10. I respect women who place their children for adoption.

Think about what your answers mean to you. You may want to discuss your thinking with your partner, someone in your family, a trusted friend, or your counselor.

sent them *and* you. If you choose independent adoption, you should consider having a lawyer of your own. To find one, contact your local state bar association, Family Court, local family service organization, or Legal Aid Society. A social worker can also help you find a lawyer.

You will be asked to sign a "take into care" form after you give birth. This allows the adoptive parents to take the child home while the state studies their family life and home environment. The study takes six to eight weeks. During this time, either you or the prospec-

Foster Care

In some cities and counties, temporary foster care may be available for the children of mothers who need more time to decide between adoption and parenting.

You and the child's birth father must both sign a legal foster care agreement to have another family care for your child. It's a good idea to consider a legal contract even if someone in your family provides the foster care. Legal contracts can help prevent misunderstandings.

Foster care agreements include:
- how often you agree to visit your child
- how long your child will stay with the foster care family
- how much money you may have to pay for the child's care
- how often you must see the social worker

You could lose your rights to your child if you don't keep your part of the agreement. It is important to remember that foster care is only temporary and is not a good substitute for a permanent home.

Laws about foster care vary from state to state. To find out more about foster care, consult your state's department of child welfare or talk with someone at the Planned Parenthood health center nearest you: 800-230-PLAN.

tive parents may change your minds. When the study is over, you will be asked to sign relinquishment papers.

For information and referrals about independent adoption, call the Independent Adoption Center hotline: 800-877-OPEN. Or write to the Independent Adoption Center, 319 Taylor Blvd., Ste. 100, Pleasant Hill, CA 94523. Planned Parenthood and other family planning centers can also provide information about independent adoption. For the Planned Parenthood health center nearest you, call 800-230-PLAN.

Adoption by Relatives

You may want your child to stay in your own family. However, independent adoptions with a relative must also be approved by a family- or surrogate-court judge. Your relatives will have to be studied by a state agency before the adoption can be finalized. And you will have no more right to the child than if you had placed it with strangers.

For more information about adoption, contact the National Adoption Information Clearinghouse, 1400 "I" St., NW, Ste. 600, Washington, DC 20005; 202-842-1919. Or call your local Planned Parenthood center. For the Planned Parenthood health center nearest you, call 800-230-PLAN.

What about Abortion?

One of your choices is abortion. Induced abortion is a legal and safe medical procedure. More than 90 percent of abortions occur during the first 12 weeks of pregnancy.

There are two kinds of induced abortion:

- **Surgical abortion** is usually performed between the sixth and eighth weeks of pregnancy.
- **Medical abortion** may be performed much earlier—as soon as a pregnancy is confirmed with a pregnancy test. As we go to press, the U. S. Food and Drug Administration is expected to approve medical abortion procedures.

Vacuum aspiration is the usual method of surgical abortion. In this procedure, first the cervix is numbed, usually with a local anesthetic. Then the embryo or fetus is removed through a narrow tube with vacuum suction. It takes about five minutes and is usually done in a clinic, doctor's office, or hospital. You don't need to stay overnight. Most likely, you can return to your normal activities the next day. Surgical abortions performed later in pregnancy may be more complicated.

Medical abortion uses medication prescribed by a doctor and does not require surgery. Medical abortion must take place within the first seven weeks of pregnancy. Two combinations of medication are used for medical abortion:

- **Methotrexate-misoprostol method.** In this method, a woman receives an injection of methotrexate from her clinician. Five to seven days later, she returns and inserts suppositories of misoprostol into her vagina. The pregnancy usually ends at home within a day or two. The embryo and other tissue that develops during pregnancy are passed out through the vagina.

- **Mifepristone-misoprostol method.** In this method, a woman swallows a dose of mifepristone under the guidance of her clinician. She returns in several days and inserts suppositories of misoprostol into her vagina. The pregnancy usually ends at home within four hours. The embryo and other tissue that develops during pregnancy are passed out through the vagina.

Abortion is one of the safest operations available. Serious complications are rare. But the risk of complications increases the longer a pregnancy continues. Most women say that early abortion feels like menstrual cramps. Other women say it feels very uncomfortable. Still others feel very little. Uncomplicated abortion should not affect future pregnancies.

If you choose abortion, you will need to sign a form that says you:

- have been *informed* about all your options
- have been *counseled* about the procedure, its risks, and how to care for yourself afterward
- have *chosen* abortion of your own free will

Most teenagers consult their parents before an abortion. Many states require that a woman under the age of 18 tell a parent or get a parent's permission, if the woman cannot talk with her parents, or chooses not to, she can speak with a judge in court. The judge will decide whether she is mature enough to make her own decision about abortion. If the judge finds that she is not mature enough, the judge will decide if abortion is in her best interest. Find out about the law in your state. Your local Planned Parenthood can help you with this process.

Most women feel relieved after an abortion. Some experience anger, regret, guilt, or sadness for a short time. These feelings may be complicated by the abrupt hormonal changes that take place after abortion. Serious, long-term emotional problems after abortion are rare. They are more likely to occur after childbirth.

You are more likely to experience serious regrets after abortion if you have strong religious feelings against it or if you have been pressured or forced into having the procedure. Be sure to examine your moral concerns before choosing abortion. Counseling is available before and after abortion.

Some doctors perform abortions in their offices during the first 12 weeks of pregnancy. Most large cities and many smaller communities have abortion providers. Look in the Yellow Pages under "abortion." Abortions are also available in many Planned Parenthood health centers, and in many other reproductive health clinics and in hospitals. For the Planned Parenthood health center nearest you, call 800-230-PLAN.

Ask beforehand about payment. Some providers want to be paid in advance. Some accept credit cards. Sometimes installment plans can be worked out. Some insurance covers part or all of the cost. In *all* states, Medicaid will pay for abortion if the woman's life is in danger. In *some* states, Medicaid will pay for abortion for other reasons, too. Check with your local Planned Parenthood center or your state or local health or welfare department for the kind of Medicaid coverage in your state.

Here are some things to consider if you are thinking about abortion:

True False

[ ]   [ ]   1. No one is pressuring me to choose abortion.

[ ]   [ ]   2. I have strong religious beliefs against abortion.

[ ]   [ ]   3. I look down on women who have abortions.

[ ]   [ ]   4. I'd rather have a child at another time.

[ ]   [ ]   5. I can afford to have another child.

[ ]   [ ]   6. I can afford to have an abortion.

[ ]   [ ]   7. I care about what other people will think.

[ ]   [ ]   8. I can handle the abortion experience.

[ ]   [ ]   9. I'll go before a judge if necessary.

[ ]   [ ]   10. I would do anything to end this pregnancy.

Think about what your answers mean to you. You may want to discuss your thinking with your partner, someone else in your family, a trusted friend, or your counselor.

You can get abortion information and assistance at Planned Parenthood and other family planning centers, women's health centers, youth centers, and departments of health or social services. Or you can call the National Abortion Federation hotline: 800-772-9100.

Afterword

"When a woman is faced with a sexual or reproductive decision, I cannot for the life of me see that anyone but that woman has the right to decide what she's going to do. That's what the birth control movement is all about...

The people who deeply worry me are the minority who wish to force us all to live according to their rules...We must oppose them— with the same courage with which my parents and Margaret Sanger opposed the moralistic repressionists of their day.

The world... is filled with wild injustices that cry out to be rectified. That's what Planned Parenthood has been struggling to do, for three generations—to ensure a decent existence and a healthy, self-empowered life for every woman and man. I cherish the freedom of choice that has allowed me to shape my life. Why should any individual, anywhere, have anything less?"

—Katharine Hepburn

Index

Note: Bracketed items denote pages on which tables and figures appear.